American Medical Association
Physicians dedicated to the health of America

Communicating with Your Patients

Christine A. Hinz

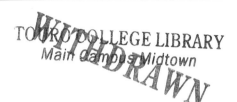

Skills for

Building

Rapport

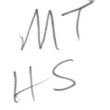

Communicating with Your Patients
Skills for Building Rapport

Additional copies of this book may be ordered by calling toll-free 800 621-8335.
Mention product number OP 208999.

ISBN 0-89970-973-7

BP37:98-1296:2.5M:12/99

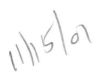

Preface

Perhaps the greatest gift we have as human beings is our ability to communicate with each other. Not only is communication fundamental to all our worldly achievements, it also enables us to connect with each other in life's more mysterious ways. What better way to address both the art *and* science of medicine than to respect the power of communication in these very different, but equally important, realms? Whether it be in the realm of the worldly or the mysterious, the more empathic the communication, the more effective the results.

The fact that our language is as subtle as it is specific allows us to convey the many complexities found in patient care. Yet human communication also goes beyond mere words. These nonverbal messages play an equally important role in what we "tell" our patients about their health.

This book not only addresses the many forms of communication, it also addresses the myriad situations physicians face every day—with myriad patients. From the age-old challenge of how to break bad news to the contemporary concept of cultural competency, we present within these chapters the latest thinking on how today's physician can best cope with any number of communication challenges.

Acknowledgments

The author of this book is Christine A. Hinz, an award-winning Milwaukee, Wisconsin–based writer. She has 25 years of experience in health care journalism, including creating and managing *Life in Medicine*, a magazine for physicians, and writing for both consumer and physician-oriented publications.

Special thanks to Geoff Gordon, MD, Associate Director of The Bayer Institute for Health Care Communications, for his invaluable assistance in the development and review of the manuscript. Dr Gordon identified numerous concepts, resources, and other people, all of which helped to make this book a valuable tool for physicians. The Bayer Institute is a noncommercial, nonprofit organization whose mission is to improve health care through education, research, and advocacy in the area of clinician-patient communication.

The following people also made significant contributions to this book. Their efforts are both acknowledged and appreciated.

Michael J. Scotti, Jr, MD
Vice President
Medical Education Group
American Medical Association

Suzanne Fraker
Director
Product Line Development
Book and Product Group
American Medical Association

Jean Roberts
Managing Editor
Product Line Development
Book and Product Group
American Medical Association

Karla Powell
Freelance Developmental Editor

Patrick Dati
Marketing Manager
Sales and Marketing
Book and Product Group
American Medical Association

Selby Toporek
Senior Communications Coordinator
Marketing Services
Book and Product Group
American Medical Association

Donald Frye
Senior Print Coordinator
Marketing Services
Book and Product Group
American Medical Association

Contents

Chapter 1

An Overview of Patient-Physician Communications

Few things you do as a physician are as important as communicating with your patients. After all, your ability to interact with individuals can have a profound effect on how they do—and on how they perceive you. Is it as a competent *and* compassionate clinician?

Even if connecting with people was the reason you entered medicine, you may be ill prepared for the task. For all the goodwill you have toward patients, there's a good chance that communicating effectively with them was the missing link in your training. Granted medical school and residency taught you the intricacies of interviewing. Yet there's more to interacting with patients than taking detailed histories and thinking good thoughts. Compassion and concern have characterized the patient-physician relationship for centuries. But only recently has research quantified the impact of certain skills—empathy and communication for starters— on a person's emotional and physiological well-being. Physicians who master these qualities build therapeutic relationships that produce satisfied patients.

But building these relationships takes a special mind-set. In this scenario, clinicians invite individuals to actively participate in their care. They encourage patients to tell their stories and express their emotions. And they share the conversation and decision making so that before the encounter is over, they've found common ground from which to deal with the problem.

In short, when physicians are empathetic, they're prepared to look into their patient's world and, with that person, craft a shared understanding of his or her disease. When they combine genuine interest with good communication skills, they have a potent intervention that reaps rewards, not just for patients, but for themselves as well. As Jenni Levy, MD, assistant professor of clinical medicine at Pennsylvania State University College of Medicine, observes:

> Many doctors do themselves a disservice. They don't think carefully enough or are not aware of the impact of what they say. So they present themselves as uncaring when they're not. I don't know very many physicians who are truly uncaring. But I know many who've come across that way because they just don't know how to help people understand that they're listening.

Managing Time in Managed Care

Time management—therein lies the biggest communication challenge. How do you develop a healthy relationship with your patients when managed care is hovering overhead, shortening visits, interrupting continuity, or even eroding the trust you're trying to build? What skills are necessary to build and maintain bonds with individuals?

Unfortunately, there are so many variations on the managed care theme that your experience may bear little resemblance to that of your colleagues elsewhere. You may find that because you're tethered to such a tight schedule, you're robbed of essential time to educate patients no matter what you attempt. Or you're micromanaged to the point that while 8 minutes may be fine for a hypertension check, it is nowhere near long enough to address a more complex topic. Maybe you trained in a managed care environment where efficiency and economy were so important that you learned how to squeeze every morsel from 15 minutes. Or perhaps the plan you're currently under leaves you to decide for yourself how long you'll take with each visit.

No matter what the appointment book throws your way, you can be an effective communicator even if you think that you have more to cover in less time. That doesn't mean you have to work faster; you just have to work differently. That is, you can't rely on the traditional physician-centered interview as your sole source of information. It may seem efficient in gathering data because it usually focuses quickly on someone's symptoms. But it can be surprisingly inefficient. By singling out only bits of a history, as one expert suggests, "like picking wildflowers from a field," you can miss the real source of someone's discomfort.

Instead, reorder your communication priorities to hear your patient first, and you streamline the interview to tackle the real problem at hand. The result is a more fruitful encounter, in which you encourage your patient to speak up as well as listen. Writing in the December 1995 issue of the *Western Journal of Medicine*, Geoffrey Gordon, MD, and colleagues suggest that good communication skills can help clinicians create and maintain healthy relationships—even in a managed care environment.

For starters, physicians ensure that individuals "feel heard" without sacrificing efficiency when they remember the simple courtesies: Sit down, make eye contact, and remove any physical barriers. They let patients know that their issues are important when they invite individuals to finish their opening statements without interrupting. And they ensure that the most serious symptoms and issues of their patients take center stage by asking them to "put all their cards on the table" up-front so they're not waiting until the last minutes of the visit.

The likely consequence of this behavior is a more satisfied patient who doesn't feel rushed because his or her essential needs are being met. Added to that are multiple other spin-offs: Outcomes improve. Compliance is better. Patients are more eager to modify their health behaviors and less eager, when the opportunity exists, to bring suit. In fact, studies repeatedly show that people have better blood pressure and diabetic control when they participate more actively in their care.

Likewise, the medical literature is replete with data linking patient dissatisfaction and the decision to sue with a lack of empathy and failure to communicate caring. In the June 27, 1994, issue of the *Archives of Internal Medicine*, for example, author Howard R. Beckman, MD, and colleagues found relationship issues prompting litigation in 71% of malpractice lawsuit depositions. Litigants repeated several common themes involving physicians: perceived unavailability, poor delivery of information, and repeated failure to understand their concerns or those of their families.

Given that message, you have all the more reason to make the most of your interview. When both of you are less hurried, there's a greater likelihood that each of you will leave the encounter satisfied and with a sense of completion. Moreover, you may even experience less discomfort or pressure when you have to add patients to your schedule or move to the next appointment. As one expert notes:

> A good communicator can make patients feel that they're the center of attention and that they understand and are getting to the heart of the matter fairly quickly. A poor communicator can have an hour and it still doesn't help.

Tuning Tin Ears

"Listen to the patient," wrote Sir William Osler, the 19th century medical thinker. "He's telling you the diagnosis." Other experts would add the word *actively*. For listening attentively means showing interest by encouraging patients to share in the discussion and participate in the decision making.

Some studies suggest that patients have at least three concerns when they come to the office, even though none of them may get heard. Other experts postulate that for every stated complaint, there's an unstated anxiety. The first brings the patient in to see the physician, but the second needs to be addressed for the person to feel satisfied with the encounter.

But physicians often aren't tuned into the latter. Two studies, in particular, reveal that while physicians are improving, they still let little time elapse at the beginning of the encounter before switching the direction of the conversation. According to a study by Howard Beckman, MD, and colleagues published in the November 1984 issue of the *Annals of Internal Medicine*, it took clinicians just 18 seconds before they interrupted patients. Only 2% of those individuals returned to their original agenda. Instead, most physicians went forth, not knowing what their patients wanted to discuss. Fifteen years later, a second study chronicled a similar experience, even though the interval cited in the January 20, 1999, *Journal of the American Medical Association (JAMA)*, by M. Kim Marvel, PhD, and colleagues had increased to 23 seconds.

Other research, including a review of studies by Moira Stewart, PhD, in the May 1, 1995, *Canadian Medical Association Journal*, reveals that 54% of patient problems and 45% of their concerns are missed in the interaction because they're neither elicited by physicians nor offered by patients. Further, in 50% of visits, parties don't agree on the presented problem. At the same time, 50% of psychiatric and psychological problems are missed.

You may think you understand what's rattling someone's cage—for example, the classic headache that must be a brain tumor. But in reality this person's agenda might not be so obvious because his or her concerns are based on a model that you don't share.

For instance, when your female patient reports that she bumped her breast and has pain, it helps to know that she comes from a culture where women believe breast cancer is caused by trauma. The information gives you a heads up that your patient might be worried enough about the possibility that you need to reassure her everything is fine. As Levy observes:

> You walk a fine line. I don't want to denigrate their concerns, so I try not to say to people, "This isn't serious." I try to say, "I understand this is a real issue for you and I'm going to help you with it. But I want you to know it's not dangerous or life threatening."

At any rate, you want to create a framework in which it is possible for that conversation to occur. By using a *biopsychosocial* approach to your interview, you're able to judge someone's health status based on the many physical, psychological, and social characteristics—personality traits and cultural beliefs, family support and community ties, job situation and financial status—that shape his or her persona.

This approach promotes the kinds of mutual discussions on which physicians can build partnerships with patients over many tasks: choosing treatments, discussing prognoses, and outlining prevention. It relies on the integrated patient-centered interview, a model that utilizes many of the skills—closed-ended questions for starters—that you've known since training. But in this model your initial task is to focus entirely on your patient's concerns: "How are things?" or "What brings you here today?" or "What are the most important concerns you want to address before you leave today?"

No interruptions. No bias. The information flows freely until the person has provided every relevant detail. As you can see, your focus isn't isolated on specific symptoms in anticipation of certain diagnoses, treatments, or advice. Instead, you're viewing this individual's problem in a larger context by encouraging him or her to share beliefs, preferences, experiences, and fears.

"Physicians hear the first couple of cues of what possibly could be wrong and they're off and running, trying to fit them into a diagnostic profile," says Barbara F. Shars, PhD, professor of humanities in medicine and speech and communication, Texas A&M University. "But, in so doing, they cut off potentially valuable information.

"If they take the first cue the patient throws out and don't hear the rest, their time may not be spent in an effective way. They think that they're saving a few seconds but they may be wasting all their minutes."

Art in Asking

There's a finesse in moving the interview along. In his book, *The Patient's Story*, Robert C. Smith, MD, professor of psychiatry and medicine at Michigan State University, suggests that among the various facilitating skills, silence, nonverbal encouragement, and neutral utterances urge patients to keep talking. When you're quiet for 5- or 10-second intervals, for instance, you force a patient to fill the void. You'll know by a shift in the person's eyes or position when the pauses are uncomfortable and you need to switch to nonverbal cues: a sympathetic expression, a rotary motion of the hand, or a change in your body language to lean forward. Utterances such as "Oh," "Uh-huh," "Yes," or "Mmm" also keep things moving.

Similarly, Smith suggests that echoing words or phrases—"The pain?"—reinforces the fact that you're listening. Open-ended requests—"Go on" and "Tell me more"—give permission to expand or delve deeper. And summarizing signals that you've heard the message.

Although these techniques are important, they seldom give you the complete picture. Eventually, you need to move the patient to the physician-centered segment of the interview. You can make the transition simply by saying, "I appreciate you sharing these things, but we're going to have to shift gears now. I need to ask you questions about your symptoms."

Similar statements keep the patient on board while you begin to evaluate the previous information and develop new hypotheses of your own. As a complement to you previous queries, closed-ended questions clarify and enhance information, shaping your ideas and confirming your intuition: "When did the pain begin?" "Do you have shortness of breath?" or "How high was your fever?"

Not surprising, your questioning skills won't matter much if you're not tuned into to what's driving the answers. Understanding a patient's emotions is as important as anything you do, given the central role they play in someone's physical well-being. Fortunately, employing empathic skills doesn't mean you have to sacrifice the efficiency of your interview. Contrary to what physicians frequently fear, patients are often brief in their emotional expression and responsive to direction by their physicians.

In his book, Smith identifies a panoply of empathic techniques that should help you be efficient and brief in eliciting and developing those feelings. The mnemonic **NURS**, for instance, summarizes the areas you want to touch on in empathizing with your patient.

> You show that you properly recognize what's been said when you **N**ame the emotion: "That sounds sad for you."

> You acknowledge an **U**nderstanding of this patient's reaction when you respond: "Given what happened, it makes sense to me; I can sure understand why," or "I've never had that happen, but I can see how deeply it hurts."

> You exhibit **R**espect for the difficulties your patient has faced when you praise with: "You've really been through a lot," or "I like the way you've hung in there and kept fighting."

> Finally, you, **S**upport the person and show that this is a partnership when you offer: "I'm here to help in any way I can. Together, you and I can get to the bottom of this."

Talking Change

Being on the same team with your patient is particularly crucial when you want this person to change attitudes or modify behavior. Adhering to medical regimens. Reducing self-injurious habits. Promoting healthy lifestyles. All three areas can present communication challenges, especially as you integrate someone else's opinion.

But the same core interviewing skills that got you to this point should help you elicit your patient's opinion and then tailor your advice. Anything less and your suggestions will fall on deaf ears. For you can't influence attitudes if you don't continue to engage the individual in the discussion, establish a working agenda, and empathize with his or her story. (Follow the last step with education to connect current health behavior with concerns and you have four important "Es" of patient-physician communication.)

"When physicians don't have those pieces in place, then behavior change becomes pretty much advice giving—if they get into it at all," says Daniel O'Connell, MD, clinical instructor at the University of Washington School of Medicine, Seattle. "Most often, they don't get into it because they're already sensing that the patient isn't with them."

Instead, your focus should be on motivating people to reflect, long after they leave the office, on what you've just said. In fact, if better outcomes are the goal, you want to make sure this patient truly buys into your diagnosis and is confident of the game plan. Unfortunately, as nonadherence rates will show, too often physicians don't find out from the get-go if their suggestions are doable or their patients are even committed. They're not aware that this individual already is grappling with other health regimens or that person has issues—the prescriptions are too costly or the side effects too significant—too awesome to take on anything new. Instead, you can clear the air by asking:

"How confident are you, honestly, that you'll be able to do these finger sticks and change your diet so we get your diabetes under control?"

"Which of these directions will be the most difficult for you to do?" or

"Tell me, Mr Smith, how convinced are you right now that taking this medicine is essential to control your high blood pressure."

Once you know that the plan sounds good but there are too many obstacles, or the prescription seems important but is too expensive, you're better positioned to modify your course. Simplify the strategy and suggest it be implemented in stages. Provide additional resources or new therapy. Order more frequent visits and follow-up calls: "Why don't you come back in two weeks and let's see how you're doing."

You want to use the same oversight when you're dealing with patients who have self-injurious behaviors: smoking, drinking, or overeating, for example. The addictive habits may be different, but the problem—immediate short-term pleasure in exchange for later long-term consequences—are often the same. In fact, the biggest obstacle you may be dealing with in changing this person's behavior is the ambivalence he or she may have over any discomfort now to have success later.

"When you think about quitting smoking, Mr Smith, what are the thoughts that come right into your mind?" or

"When I encourage you to do a breast self-exam, Mrs Phillips, tell me what goes through your head."

The answers may quickly reveal that Mr Smith gets pleasure from smoking even though he worries about cancer and heart disease. Or Mrs. Phillips is reluctant to perform her monthly breast exam because she's clueless as to what she's feeling or frightened by the prospects. But at least you understand the motivatins and can target the advice.

"I think there has been a notion among physicians that, depending on their own psychological training, they must do psychoanalysis to understand the deep unconscious of the patient, which is not true," says O'Connell. "What they have to do is to understand the patient's current thinking."

But you don't want to argue with your patient. Debates are unproductive even though many doctors like to engage in them. An in-your-face attitude only makes patients angry and puts up roadblocks for any future discussions. After all, it's natural for people to feel alienated if you're not invested in them anymore than glancing up from the chart with a blunt assessment: "I have to tell you, Mr Smith, I don't think your chances are very good if you don't stop smoking."

Instead, it's more productive to listen attentively and confront gently, always focusing your remarks on the discrepancies between the person's behavior and what should be his or her health goals:

"This is enormously important, Mr Smith. I really hope that as we continue to work on your recovery from this heart attack, you and I can keep in the foremost part of our minds those things you're doing that are putting you more at risk." or

"Mr Brown, I have to tell you that I'm worried. On one hand, you have a family history of heart disease and a cholesterol count over 350. On the other hand, it sounds like any time I suggest a dietary change you tell me how it is impossible."

In either case, you're declaring that this behavior will only take Mr Smith or Mr Brown down a well-worn path. Similarly, if either of them confides that past attempts to quit a 35-year, two-pack-a-day habit nearly produced a nervous breakdown, empathize. But then segue into your pitch:

"Boy, it sounds like for you the addiction to smoking is enormous and the only way you will consider cutting down—let's throw away the word stop *—is if we can find some way to help you. Well, thank goodness we have a patch. We have gum. We have Wellbutrin. We have things we can do."*

If you listen for the obstacle, you open up creative possibilities. You just may be able to make your case by introducing information that frames the topic in a new way. Or maybe you can back up your advice with a bit of data, especially if what you're about to say differs greatly from what your patient believes or understands.

> *"You know, it may surprise you to learn that. . . ."*

> *"We know that wearing a helmet reduces head injuries in children who fall off their bikes by. . . ." or*

> *"It's not just important to lose some weight, but you know, Mr Brown, we've learned that regular exercise at your age has these specific benefits. . . . I really encourage you to think about that and to find where in your lifestyle you could fit it."*

While you can't always "eliminate the negative" when it comes to motivating patients, you may want to "accentuate the positive," as the old tune goes. In his book, *Real Age: Are You as Young as You Can Be?* author Michael F. Roizen, MD, suggests that patients focus on the rewards of a healthy lifestyle rather than just dwelling on the risks associated with certain unhealthy behaviors. In other words, the chairman of anesthesia and critical care at the University of Chicago Pritzger School of Medicine believes you can actually calculate how many years of healthy living any number of daily choices—exercise and a balanced diet for starters—will add to your calendar age.

Computing choices maybe a helpful hook with some patients. But it's likely you won't need a formula to drive home your lifestyle message if you've established rapport and this person already is armed with information.

When Margaret J. Byers, DO, a Milwaukee, Wisconsin, obstetrician/gynecologist, talks to women, she likes to focus on the positive because it adds a "whole new energy" to the discussion. In fact, because many of her patients are already self-advocates, she's often just updating what they know, even learning from them.

But that's not everyone. For some women, especially those with addictive behaviors, even the most compelling reasons won't make them budge. "I can quote statistics to them all day long," she says, "but until they own it, or see a personal consequence from it, they won't take the next step."

While Byers has learned to accept patients where they're at, often health concerns are so pressing that she, too, resorts to blunt talk and even written commitments. When a new pregnant patient came into her office for the first time, the physician knew she had to do more than talk to this woman about prenatal care. The young mother had a history of cocaine and nicotine abuse and was already suing another physician over the disastrous delivery of her severely disabled young son.

After asking the woman to level with her about the current litigation, Byers felt comfortable that she wasn't out to get every physician. But she went one step further than just a discussion. The two women wrote a contract that detailed both their expectations about her care. The issues were very specific: She couldn't miss her office visits. Byers would do random drug screens. There would be extra surveillance of the baby. While the woman agreed to stay away from narcotics, the physician acquiesced, as part of the give-and-take of negotiation, to her smoking a bit.

Byers doesn't write many formal contracts with patients. But in this case, committing specifics to paper turned out to be key in making change. At the end of her pregnancy, the patient delivered a healthy baby—with no disastrous results. Even better, however, was that she no longer needed drugs to deal with painful issues. Instead, with the help of a supportive partner whom she ultimately married, she saw her life come together in many positive ways.

In fact, a year later, the patient wrote Byers a wonderful note saying that she'd be forever grateful that someone had respected her as a human being and given her a chance to respect herself. It would make her, she assured the doctor, a better parent.

"I think that the way we approached it together and stated our expectations made a huge difference," she says. "Just laying the groundwork for what both of us were OK with—and knowing that someone was going to be there for her—gave her the support she needed to do it."

Obviously, Byers would have been there whether or not her patient met expectations. But by being specific up-front, she encouraged this woman to take ownership of her own health—and that of her baby. Your patient may also have a pressing reason— new onset diabetes or a near-fatal heart attack—to make immediate changes. But more often than not, it may seem that getting this patient to buy into the program is like turning the *Titanic*. As O'Connell observes: "Somebody who is steering this has to decide that little by little they want to change direction. I think the challenge is for physicians to keep at it, not in a harrying way, but to keep tailoring advice."

But the rewards are worth the patience. Building relationships and rapport over time can be particularly beneficial if your patient perceives that the managed care plan or organization governing you both doesn't have his or her best interests at heart. Or if he or she is frustrated that care has been interrupted or benefits dropped.

Gordon suggests that the same approaches you use throughout your encounter can help you through the communication dilemmas posed by managed care. Ascertain someone's opinion. Empathize with this person's frustrations. Acknowledge that the two of you may disagree on an issue. By framing the discussion and identifying or countering the feelings, you can negotiate your way through any conversation about why you can't fill this particular request, make that particular referral, or bend the rules of that particular plan.

In fact, the associate director for clinical education and research, Bayer Health Institute for Healthcare Communication, suggests that physicians keep the focus on the quality of care they can administer through the plan rather than comparing it with others. As Gordon observes:

> I think that one of the things that we don't communicate very often in managed care is to say, "Mr Jones, you have a good plan here. It lets me do the things that you need in order to treat your disease and keep you healthy. It has some limitations that you and I need to figure out. And we need to prioritize your needs so they get met. But, you know, this plan allows me to do most of what I would want to do with you."

Obviously, you want to reassure Mr Jones that if something—a referral to a specialist or a procedure that isn't covered—comes up that you both agree he needs, you'll help him get it. And you might even encourage this person to be an activist for his own health since patient-initiated appeals are often successful and individuals who flourish in managed care plans are those who take charge. At the same time, you're also prepared to warn him when, in your medical judgment, the treatment he seeks really won't help. You understand your patient's predicament, but you reiterate that he might want to consider if this procedure is truly beneficial before waging a campaign for it.

In any case, by sharing responsibility even in the most difficult of exchanges, you're empowering your patient. You're enhancing his or her sense of autonomy and feelings of support and trust. Yet you're doing something even more important for yourself. In creating a more humanistic interaction, you raise your own profile as a medically competent individual with integrity and compassion. You also create a sense of "connectedness" that some suggest is part of the spiritual dimension of medicine, and you're poised to bask in the goodwill that may have brought you into the profession in the first place.

But even more basic, by listening carefully to your patient and paying attention to your words, you ensure that even the simplest message is transmitted correctly. Edward Rosenbaum, MD, whose book *A Taste of My Own Medicine* was the basis for the movie *The Doctor,* learned an important lesson about communication when a young woman called him after her annual examination and asked "Doctor, when am I going to die?"

A stunned Rosenbaum couldn't imagine what prompted the question since he had just given his patient a stellar bill of health. But he was even more surprised when she answered: "You did. Yesterday after you completed the report on my physical examination, you walked out of the room, put your arm around me, and said, 'Good-bye old friend.' You never said that before."

Bibliography

Beckman H, Markakis K, Suchman A, Frankel R. Getting the most from a 20-minute visit. *Am J Gastroenterol.* 1994;89:662-664.

Beckman H, Markakis K, Suchman A, Frankel R. The doctor-patient relationship and malpractice: lessons from plaintiff depositions. *Arch Intern Med.* 1994;154:1365-1369.

Council on Ethical and Judicial Affairs. Ethical issues in managed care. *JAMA.* 1995;273:330-335.

Deber R, Kraetschmer N, Irvine J. What role do patients wish to play in treatment decision-making?" *Arch Intern Med.* 1996;156:1414-1420.

Enelow A, Forde D, Brummel-Smith K. *Interviewing and Patient Care.* 4th ed. New York, NY: Oxford University Press; 1996.

Frankel R. *Communicating with Patients: Research Shows It Makes a Difference.* Deerfield, Ill: MMI Risk Management Resources, Inc; 1994.

Gordon G, Baker L, Levinson W. Physician-patient communication in managed care. *West J Med.* 1995;163:527-531.

Levinson W, Roter D, Mullooly J, Dull V, Frankel R. Physician-patient communication: the relationship with malpractice claims among primary care physicians and surgeons. *JAMA.* 1997;277:553-559.

Levinson W, Stiles W, Inui T, Engle R. Physician frustration in communicating with patients. *Med Care.* 1993;31:285-295.

Lipkin M. The medical interview. In: Feldman MD, Christensen JF, eds. *Behavioral Medicine Primary Care: A Practical Guide.* Norwalk, Conn: Appleton & Lange; 1997:1-7.

Lipkin M, Putnam S, Lazare A, eds. *The Medical Interview: Clinical Care, Education, and Research.* New York, NY: Springer Publishing Company; 1995.

Marvel M, Epstein R, Flowers K, Beckman H. Soliciting the patients' agenda: have we improved? *JAMA.* 1999;281:283-287.

Mishler E. *The Discourse of Medicine.* Norwood, NJ: Ablex Publishing Corporation; 1984.

Ness D, Ende J. Denial in the medical interview. *JAMA.* 1994;272:1777-1781.

Osler W. The master-word in medicine. In: *Agequanimitas with Other Addresses to Medical Students, Nurses and Practitioners of Medicine.* Philadelphia, Pa: Blakiston; 1904.

Quill T. Partnership in patient care: a contractual approach. *Ann Intern Med.* 1983;98:228-233.

Sander R, Holloway R, Eliason B, Marbella A, Murphy B, Yuen S. Patient-initiated prevention discussions: two interventions to stimulate patients to initiate prevention discussions. *J Fam Pract.* 1996;43:468-474.

Sharf B. Physician-patient communication as interpersonal rhetoric: a narrative approach. *Health Commun.* 1990;2:217-231.

Smith RC, Engel G. *The Patient's Story.* Boston, Mass: Little, Brown & Company; 1996.

Smith R, Hoppe R. The patient's story: integrating the patient- and physician-centered approaches to interviewing. *Ann Intern Med.* 1991;115:470-475.

Spiro H. What is empathy and can it be taught? *Ann Intern Med.* 1992;116:843-846.

Stewart M. Effective physician-patient communication and health outcomes: a review. *Can Med Assoc J.* 1995;152:1423-1432.

Chapter 2

Breaking Bad News: Ease the Pain Through Empathic Communication

As patient encounters go, this one wasn't going to be a walk in the park. Ronald E. Waldridge II knew it. Here he was, a third-year medical student trapped by a resident on his internal medicine rotation into telling a young man they both had just met that he had HIV.

Granted, by this point in his training Waldridge understood the implications of the tests ordered after this patient's seizures landed him in the hospital. A CT scan was consistent with toxoplasmosis, and blood tests confirmed that he had the virus. But nothing had prepared Waldridge for breaking such news. No one had told him how to minimize the trauma, for either himself or the patient.

"I knew that it wasn't going to be a good outcome, and so I didn't relish the thought," he recalls. "I remember vividly his mother and partner anxiously awaiting the news. It was the first time I realized what a big impact it made, not just for the patient but for a whole circle of friends and family. That made it all the more uncomfortable."

Waldridge recalls little about the words that tumbled from his mouth that day except blurting, "The test came back positive for the HIV virus that causes AIDs." No measured delivery. No checks to see if the patient was ready to receive the information—or prepared for what it meant. Just a nasty diagnosis, delivered by someone who knew little more about the disease than how it is contracted and its probable outcome.

When the patient shot back his own questions—"When do I start treatment? How long do I have to live?"—Waldridge was stumped. He had few answers other than "I'll have to check that" and "I have no idea."

He was right. It was no walk in the park.

Anywhere but Here

In those few moments, Waldridge understood what other physicians have learned over time: Breaking bad news can be the most unnerving communications task in medicine. Maybe you're the trainee facing a patient for the first time with no idea of where to begin or how to close. Worse yet, you're the physician who turns the job over to the student or resident because it challenges your self-worth, reminds you of your mortality, or makes you feel like you've failed.

Indeed, there are many reasons that physicians find breaking bad news a daunting task. As a practitioner, you may be intimately familiar with many of them. Perhaps you're close to this particular patient or your parent died from that particular disease. Maybe you're anxious that family members will pose too many questions or this person will cry too much.

Conceivably, you never learned how to give hope when the message is bleak. In fact, your anxiety may be rooted in a lack of requisite skills on this topic. Your medical school never made this communication task compulsory, and you never had a role model during residency to show you how to do so.

True, on those scores you may have a legitimate complaint. But it's never too late to develop competency in an area so vital to your practice. Breaking bad news is part of the job, a task to be shared by the person who'll be there for the long haul—despite the discomfort. As John F. Christensen, PhD, director of behavioral medicine training, department of medicine, Legacy Portland Hospitals, in Oregon, and faculty member, Northwest Center for Physician-Patient Communication, observes:

> It's one of those inherent difficulties that goes with the territory of being in medicine. It's inevitable in this profession that physicians will come face to face with suffering that can't be controlled. So learning to be respectfully present to that is a challenging task— but one from which enormous personal growth arises.

Yet there are no magic bullets. Patients and their health concerns are too individual to make a one-size-fits-all formula work for everyone. Even the definition of "bad news" suggests diversity. In his book, *Breaking Bad News: A Guide for Health Care Professionals*, author Robert Buckman, MD, oncologist and associate professor of medicine at the University of Toronto, defines it as "any news that drastically and negatively alters the patient's view of his or her future." This implies that the badness depends on the gap between an individual's perception of the situation and medical reality. Furthermore, what overwhelms one person might be accepted with peace by another. What's trivial to one individual may be horrific to another.

"Bad news is always in the eyes of the beholder," Buckman says. "It's always a drastic adverse change in expectations. And you have no idea how 'bad' the news is unless you know what the expectations are."

But knowing those expectations requires that you first develop techniques to uncover them. The good news is that the tasks important in breaking bad news already have a track record in psychotherapy: Listen, empathize, and explore a patient's concerns. As anxious as physicians might be about this encounter, they're in a powerful position to provide support, says Walter F. Baile, MD, chief of psychiatry service, department of neuro-oncology at M.D. Anderson Cancer Center, Houston.

> When you respect a patient, when you sit down and actively listen and inquire as to what this person has understood and what are their concerns, you make an empathetic response. These are tremendously supportive interventions. They would seem a balance to the helplessness that doctors feel when they have to give bad news. The worst thing about it is that you also have to find some way to be supportive and that's very difficult.

It's difficult, but it's not impossible if you think of the protocol as a set of defined steps that you can learn and shape to fit your style. Buckman puts order to the process of breaking bad news with a simple mnemonic—**SPIKES**. **S** is for sharpening your listening skills and staging the talk in a conducive setting; **P** stands for paying attention to your patient's perception; **I** is for the invitation you want from the patient to discuss details; and **K**, the knowledge and facts you need to corral; **E** represents emotions you will explore and the empathy you will deliver; and **S** is the strategy you propose before summarizing your next steps.

Granted, even having a mnemonic tool is no guarantee you will master your delivery of bad news. But in changing how you approach your patient—paying closer attention to what you say and how you say it—you're bound to create a more satisfying experience for you both. Once you learn the skills, you can avoid the seemingly small errors—failing to acknowledge your patient's expectations for starters—that often lead to big blunders for physicians. By retooling certain tasks and being aware of the consequences of others you can create a less agonizing experience for everyone. As Buckman's book reminds physicians: "An expert in breaking bad news is not someone who gets it right every time. She or he is merely someone who gets it wrong less often, and who is less flustered when things do not go smoothly."

Taking a First Step

Time and place are particularly important when it comes to sharing bad news. Obviously, some medical situations don't allow the luxury of laying groundwork far in advance of such a talk. But remember the adage, "To be forewarned is to be forearmed." Having a preliminary discussion with your patient about the delivery of important medical information—as part of your routine care—can provide insight into how he or she wants to receive a diagnosis, particularly of a life-threatening condition. You could couch this talk by asking:

> *"Are you a person who wants to hear everything, or is there somebody else you'd prefer I talk to?"*

> *"Do you want a general outline of what's going on, or should I provide you all of the details?"*

Then later, if your suspicions prompt you to order a test, don't waste an opportunity to warn your patient of the possibilities in advance of the results. Physicians frequently forget that bad news discussions should begin at the time a test is ordered.

"Many physicians are either unwilling or unable to say, 'The reason I'm ordering this test is because I have some concern that what you're experiencing may be bad and I want to rule out that possibility,'" says Richard Frankel, PhD, professor of medicine at the University of Rochester School of Medicine and Dentistry. "Instead, they'll say they want to spare a patient suffering until they get the test results. If it's bad news, they'll deal with it then. But in point of fact, that's unfair to the patient."

An early warning at least plants the seed from which your next conversation can grow. Also, asking your patient to return for a follow-up visit won't bias him or her about the results one way or the other. Rather, whether the news is good or bad, it guarantees a face-to-face encounter. Also, if you have a high suspicion that the results might be positive, eg, a breast biopsy likely will show malignancy, you also can suggest early on that this person bring someone along. You can mention that you hope there will be nothing more to say. But if the two of you have to deal with anything, it might be good to have a third party hear the discussion.

"We don't know how much information patients absorb," Baile says. "In fact, studies show that they often overestimate the favorability of news transmitted by the physician. One of the reasons may be that they don't hear. Another may be that to maintain their internal hope meter high, they tend to frame it in more favorable light."

Beyond clarifying the conversation, the presence of a third party also suggests that breaking bad news should be done in person. True, you may be forced at times to deliver the report over the phone. Your patient may live far away or is commuting between countries. Or you still may be reacting to the news yourself and may not feel ready to face the patient. But nothing substitutes for the immediacy and intimacy of an eye-to-eye encounter.

A recent study suggests that patients perceive their physicians as less helpful if they disclose the information over the phone. In the May 1989 *Journal of Clinical Oncology*, author Stuart E. Lind, MD, and colleagues reported that the site of such a conversation had a bearing on how cancer patients, in particular, reacted to their diagnosis. A significantly greater percentage of persons who heard the report over the telephone or in the recovery room expressed negative feelings.

While it sounds simple, getting the physical context right puts you in control and shows your patient you know what you're doing. So sit, don't stand. Remove any barriers—furniture or family members—between you and the patient. Always make eye contact and be open to touch (eg, nonthreatening contact with a shoulder or hand) if you're invited to and are comfortable in doing so.

Your image as an empathetic healer will take a hit if your body language sends a different message. Perhaps you know someone who still has a "get out of Dodge" mentality about breaking bad news. Perhaps you're the one keeping one hand on the door and eyes fixated on the clock. In reality, you're just putting distance between yourself and your patient.

Actions speak louder than words, and your behavior can communicate volumes about your own feelings. You may think, "This is really hard and I would rather be out of here because it's too painful to do." Those are legitimate thoughts. But the challenge is to reserve dealing with your angst for another time and, in this moment, focus only on your patient.

"It's quite possible that trauma is in every interview, but with bad news it is quite likely that it's inescapable," says Buckman. "It's your job, as a healthcare professional, to support the patient while he or she is receiving the bad news.

"The objective is to put some space between the messenger and the message. You want to look after the patient, even though the message is perceived as horrible. You don't want to be identified with the information itself. You don't want to be, as it were, the Egyptian slave executed because he brings the message to Cleopatra that the battle was lost."

Dialogue Creates Exchange

A physician's ability to communicate well on this topic depends entirely on what he or she says and on how he or she says it. Physicians are most effective in disclosing diagnostic or prognostic information if they rely on the give-and-take of a dialogue, especially when it comes to bad news.

First, it allows every physician to find out how much someone may already know or even wants to know but is too anxious to ask. For example, putting up MRI results when the patient doesn't really want to know how much the tumor has grown could be distressing. As Buckman notes, "Before you tell, ask."

Second, this technique invites patients to participate. A well-placed pause or nod can be the green light your patient is waiting for to pick up the conversation. Likewise, open questions such as "How are you? " or "What did that make you feel?" may unearth a trove of real concerns.

Third, dialogue creates a structure in which both people can deal with the trauma. While a patient will no doubt need support, this can be a harrowing experience for the physician, too, especially since he or she is altering someone's view of himself or herself from "I am a healthy person" to "I am a sick or dying person."

"Sometimes it feels like you're doing something harmful because you're giving somebody something that they don't want," says Timothy Quill, MD, professor of medicine and psychiatry at the University of Rochester School of Medicine and Dentistry. "Even though they may know it's coming, it's hard because they're changing their conception of self in a way that they don't particularly want."

While hearing bad news is upsetting, the alternative—putting it off until later—is far worse. If you don't deliver important information in a timely fashion, you risk the ire of an individual (not to mention his or her attorneys). Also, it's bogus to believe that by withholding a diagnosis or prognosis, you're relieving someone's discomfort. Compassion is a useful quality for physicians—you're not going to be a very good one if you don't feel it with each patient—but it should never be a substitute for straight talk. As Buckman notes:

> What is not permissible is to avoid giving important information on the grounds, almost always spurious, that you are thereby protecting this person from damage. That's an excuse used by people who don't know how to break bad news well or break it at all. It's dangerous to think, "Oh, I can't tell him it's cancer. The shock would kill him." The shock will not kill him if you know how to tell him the bad news supportively. So compassion must never be used as an excuse to lie."

Instead, truth must drive every word you say. The first basic rule of breaking bad news is to never tell a lie. Anything else can cause a mother lode of legal and other consequences. The good news, of course, is that studies show that a majority of patients—as high as 97%—want to know their diagnosis, even though it's less clear what they expect in terms of a prognosis.

At the same time, research suggests a profession that has changed its own attitudes about delivering painful truths. Reported two decades apart in the *Journal of the American Medical Association*, two studies documented a major shift in thinking among physicians in regards to a patient's right to know if he or she has a serious condition. While 90% of practitioners interviewed by Donald Oken, MD, and colleagues in 1961 said they preferred not to reveal a cancer diagnosis, by 1979,

97% of those responding to the same questionnaire, presented by Dennis H. Novack, MD, and colleagues, would share the news.

Today, invigorated by patient protections such as informed consent, physicians generally hold that all mentally competent persons have ethical, moral, and legal rights to information. Granted, telling the truth doesn't take the "bad" out of bad news or rescue patients from the facts. But it does lay the foundation for the unpleasant tasks that follow.

As Ned H. Cassem, MD, editor of the Massachusetts General Hospital *Handbook of General Psychiatry*, observes: "Truth-telling is no panacea. Communicating a diagnosis honestly, though difficult, is easier than the labors that lie ahead. Telling the truth is merely a way to begin; but since it is an open and honest way, it provides a firm basis on which to build a relationship of trust."

An Invitation to RSVP

The challenge then becomes one of presenting the truth at a rate and in the order of priorities that this patient can handle. Give the information too abruptly, suggests Peter Maguire, FRCPsych, and an individual may have difficulty adapting or simply deny the facts as too painful to assimilate. "The key," he writes in the October 8, 1998, *British Medical Journal*, "is to try to slow down the speed of the transition from a patient's perception of himself or herself as being well to a realization that he or she has a life-threatening disease."

Indeed, a dialogue helps physicians present facts in such a way and at such a pace that a patient can decide what he or she wants to hear and when. In fact, the most critical steps you take with an individual, both initially and throughout your encounter, will be in determining his or her readiness for what comes next and then tailoring your response to fit.

Since some time has probably elapsed since the previous appointment, you'll want to establish what this person has been thinking and feeling. This is where your skills as an interrogator and good listener really begin. After the courtesies of "How are you doing?" you might launch into any number of questions that pave the way for discussion:

"Since we last spoke have you had any thoughts about your symptoms?"

"Have you been worried about what this illness might be?"

"Are you concerned that it's serious?"

Much ground already has been covered if a man confirms for you his family physician's concern that this might be multiple sclerosis. Conversely, you're starting from scratch if a woman is thankful that the breast lump the surgeon found is a "lesion" and not a "tumor" or "cancer."

In either case, listen to the words but also watch the body language—a back hunched forward or a head slumped back—as it, too, sends a powerful message. While the voice may suggest calm bravery, the hand-wringing could be signaling unleashed anxiety. By aligning with your patient, adds Quill, you may discover what wasn't obvious at first: The depth of his or her angst goes well beyond "I'm so scared" to "If it's cancer, I'm going to take the bridge." With that insight, you know you have much to do before even mentioning the diagnosis.

Just as one patient may test your skills of perception, another will help you out by saying, "Stop beating around the bush. Let's just get through it." With that kind of overture, you know this person is ready to move on to the diagnosis and you can follow immediately with your opening assessment: "I'm sorry to say that what you and I feared is the case. The biopsy shows it's cancer."

If there still seems to be some hesitancy, lead simply with "This does appear to be more serious than we thought." Or you may even review the events—the symptoms, tests, and procedures—that brought you both here. Waldridge was beyond medical school when he used such an approach with a 40-year-old mother about the CT scan of her brain that showed multiple metastases of breast cancer.

The woman had received promising prognoses after two mastectomies and follow-up rounds of chemotherapy. But when severe headaches brought her back into Waldridge's office, she agreed that the symptoms should be checked, even though she linked them to depression. When the CT scans came back, Waldridge scheduled an appointment and softened the impending blow by first reviewing the events.

> *"Remember when you came in with the headaches and I wanted to do further testing because we thought it could be related to a sinus infection? But we were also concerned that with your history of cancer there could be something causing them? That's why I ordered the CT scan. Well, it shows some areas in the brain that aren't normal. They appear to be tumors. The most likely cause of tumors of this nature is cancer spread from some other point. Like breast cancer."*

By pausing periodically in his delivery, Waldridge gave his patient time to acknowledge each development while he created a springboard to talk about the tumors found with the CT scan. By pacing the conversation and giving information in small chunks (no more than two or three sentences at a time), he could watch her grasp the meaning of every piece. "I just can't believe that I'm hearing what you're saying. I just never thought I'd have to hear this again."

Remember, from the diagnosis to its implications, each fragment of news may have a profound impact on your patient, especially if his or her self-image and worldview are threatened. In fact, some studies suggest that physicians would be well served to switch the order of information. Australian researcher Philip Ley, in particular, showed that patients are more likely to recall their prognosis rather than their diagnosis.

Medical information is hard to digest, and medical jargon is designed only to transmit data efficiently and precisely between medical colleagues. So relying on "Medspeak"—*blast cells* for leukemia or *demyelination* when it's actually multiple sclerosis—only fogs the conversation and obliterates your message. Instead, keep it simple and straightforward: Abnormal growths are tumors and the prognosis is never guarded. The situation is serious. When the doctor in a vignette proposed by Buckman told a 23-year-old woman what her bone marrow test revealed, he simplified the information by saying:

> *"Well, it told us just what is going wrong and that it's going wrong in the bone marrow. The disease is called acute myeloid leukemia. That's a bit like a sort of malignancy or a kind of a cancer in the bone marrow, and that's why you've been feeling so ill, and that's why you had the sore throat. . . ."*

Similarly, Maguire suggests that using a "hierarchy of euphemisms" for a word such as *cancer* also can be effective in managing the transition for a patient. For example:

Doctor: "I'm afraid it's more than an ulcer."

Mr K: "What do you mean more than just an ulcer?"

Doctor: "Some of the cells looked abnormal under the microscope."

Mr K: "Abnormal?"

Doctor: "They looked cancerous."

Mr K: "You mean I've got cancer?"

Doctor: "I'm afraid so, yes."

Keep in mind that people attach complex meanings to such words as *malignancy, HIV,* and *AIDS,* so it's dangerous to assume that you and your patient are on common ground until you explore it together. Any miscue can lead to disastrous consequences, as illustrated by this story of the young man who dies at the hospital after a crash. Failing to save his life, the physician tells his mother: "Unfortunately, we were unsuccessful. May we have your permission to do an autopsy?" She agrees, only to inquire later, "Was it successful?" Apocryphal? Perhaps. But this experience crystallizes how miscues can turn tragic when the message isn't understood. Clarity is as important as well-placed silence. Once you've delivered the news, repeat the essential elements and use diagrams or any other written resources to explain each point. Again, check your progress with such questions as "Am I making sense?" "Do you see what I mean?" and "Do you follow what I'm saying?"

Also, don't fill the vacuum created as the message resonates with what Frankel calls "doctor babble." Rambling, no matter how natural it seems, comes with a price. It can set up a situation in which you believe this person is hearing each word when in fact he or she hasn't retained a syllable. You leave the encounter believing that you're both singing from the same song sheet, and one of you hasn't even heard the tune. Even more confounding, you may perceive at your next visit that the patient is in denial, whereas he or she actually is ill informed, never having even heard what you said.

"Silence is a gift," Frankel says. "It allows your patients to integrate the news, at least initially. It's the point at which you give control of the interview to them and follow their lead rather than leading yourself. Unfortunately, many physicians start talking because their own feelings are stirred. They just don't know what to do."

How Does This Leave You Feeling?

Fortunately, responding empathetically doesn't require that you experience a patient's angst or agree with his or her assessment of the situation. It just demands that you listen for the obvious reactions, probe for the not so obvious, and then be led by individual concerns wherever they take you. As Buckman writes, empathy is not a matter of what you *feel*. It's a matter of how you *behave*. For example, once he delivered the diagnosis, the physician in Maguire's vignette immediately turned his attention to the reaction. Using simple cues, he elicited each response, thereby unleashing the concerns frightening this patient.

> *Doctor:* "How does this news leave you feeling?"
>
> *Mr K:* "Terrified! I've always had this thing about cancer. I've always been frightened of getting it. Two of my uncles died of it. They both had a bad time. Suffered terrible pain and wasted away to nothing."
>
> *Doctor:* "So you're frightened you're going to go the same way."
>
> *Mr K:* "I'm bound to be scared, aren't I?"
>
> *Doctor:* "Yes, you are in view of those experiences. It must be hard for you. Any other reasons you are terrified?"
>
> *Mr K:* "I hate being a burden. My wife has enough to contend with."

While Mr K worried about being a burden, your patient may be focused on the side effects of future treatment or the past experiences of friends who suffered the same condition. For the concerns patients raise about their situation are as varied as the reactions they exhibit under such stress. Those reactions depend on the meaning this person places on the diagnosis, as well as his or her previous experience with the illness and the degree of immediate threat to his or her life.

When Quill told a devoutly Christian patient that her estranged husband—an IV drug user—had infected her with the HIV virus, he was confronted by her overwhelming perception that this was a death sentence and she was now a pariah. He acknowledged, writing in the March 1991 *Archives of Internal Medicine*, that each of her perceptions contained both truth and distortion and then set about to correct any misconceptions.

> *Patient:* "I don't even have a future. Everything I know is that you gonna die anytime. What is there to do? What if I'm a walking time bomb? People will be scared to even touch me or say anything to me."

> *Dr Quill:* "No, that's not so."

> *Patient:* "Yes, they will, 'cause I feel that way about people. You don't know what to say to them and what to do. Oh God."

> *Dr Quill:* "What we have to do is to learn some things about it . . . even though it's scary it may not be as scary as you think."

Quill had to work hard during their encounter as she dealt with the news. Like this woman, patients who face threatening diagnoses are likely to call on various behavioral and emotional coping strategies including acceptance, blame, denial, disbelief, and intellectualization, along with anger (rage), anxiety, fear (terror), guilt, helplessness, hopelessness, relief, and shame.

In addition, the stress may trigger one of two other mechanisms that either leave them numb to the news, with little recollection of the discussion, or put them in motion, raging with a mix of feelings. Quill's patient, for instance, paced the floor of the small examination room, unable to sit, fearful and fuming rage against God and her husband.

> *Patient:* "Oh my God. Oh my God. I hate him. I hate him. I hate the ground he walks on. I hate him, Dr Quill. I hate him. He gave this to me. I hate him. He took my life away from me. I have been robbed. I feel as if I have been robbed of a future. I don't have nothing."

Quill gave her room to rant, fearing that if she fled she would harm herself or be alone without direction when her "high-energy state" wore off. By being allowed to express herself, she eventually accepted information that helped her put the loss into perspective and devise a follow-up plan.

While the reactions of this woman were unmistakably powerful, the response of another patient may be far more subtle. You may be dealing with someone who becomes acutely anxious or is driven by feelings of helplessness—there's nothing he or she can do—or hopelessness—there's nothing that anyone else can do. Yet another individual may just ask for the medical facts and take his or her emotions elsewhere.

In any case, your role is to identify the response, determine if it's appropriate, and then help make necessary adjustments. If you think you're out of your league, don't be afraid to get a second opinion or make a referral to a psychiatrist or other therapist. Don't count on this person's past experience to predict present behavior. While a patient's responses are rooted in how he or she has dealt with previous stresses, the picture often changes when the threat involves a life-ending illness. Something so overwhelming may lead to more intense reactions.

Also, inappropriate versions of many responses can either crop up initially or remain obscured until later. Watch for the anger that deteriorates into prolonged rage, the lifetime ambition that's suddenly replaced by an impossible quest, or the realistic expectations exchanged for unrealistic hopes.

Denial, for instance, can be healthy when it helps a patient adjust to the diagnosis. It's unhealthy when it becomes an impediment to that person moving on. The woman who focuses on her oncologist's optimism about chemotherapy and not on the surgeon's diagnosis of inflammatory breast cancer is using normal denial. When she negates reality entirely—she doesn't have cancer—that denial turns pathological.

"Honest communication of the diagnosis (or any truth) by no means precludes later avoidance or even denial of the truth," Cassem writes, citing, for example, three studies in which 20% of patients explicitly told that they had either cancer or a myocardial infarction later denied their condition. "For a person to function effectively, truth's piercing voice must occasionally be muted or even excluded from awareness."

But that exclusion is only good so long as it doesn't hinder your patient's progress or put his or her care in peril. In fact, you may need to intervene, gently but firmly, with the truth if this person seems deeply preoccupied with shutting out the information or if you see important decisions looming. Also, keep in mind that someone who wasn't prepared for a bad news diagnosis on Monday may be ready by Friday. Always leave the door open for a change of heart by suggesting, "If you want any questions answered at future visits, you just ask me. Otherwise, I won't push information at you."

Summing Up with Strategy and Support

Setting up a strategy and helping your patient continue to move forward is the final step in a bad news interview. Before your patient leaves the office, you'll want to set up a short-term plan, eg, "Call me with any questions and let's make sure you have an appointment scheduled," as well as the preliminaries of a longer-term strategy.

If your patient isn't ready for the particulars, you may have to plan for a second session to discuss tactics. If this is an emergency—he or she is having a heart attack and needs a clot buster immediately—you'll be forgoing any big-picture discussions. But if the illness doesn't necessitate immediate intervention, you'll have time to explore the options. If your patient is engaged in the discussion, you can outline the general plan and even talk specifics.

In any case, don't trap yourself into thinking that you need a thorough grasp of every disease, particularly one that you don't see much or that isn't part of your field. That reasoning may make you reluctant to take the first step. Instead, learn the basics and then be confident enough to admit when you are stumped, simply saying, "I don't know, but we'll find out." Even with limited experience, Waldridge knew instinctively that day during training that he had to punt when it came to the particulars about HIV. Today, he not only lassos the facts but also hits the high points before his patient leaves the office. Then, after that individual has seen the specialist (if one is required), he touches base with both of them to make sure his patient is clear about the treatment plan.

As Waldridge learned, information about treatment must be delivered with the same clarity as the diagnosis. In outlining the treatment for his patient, one doctor wrote the plan—chemotherapy, cisplatin 5-FU, 5 weeks, every Thursday, followed by radiation therapy—on the paper covering the examination table and gave it to her to tack on her kitchen wall.

Whatever you do, again, tell it like it is. When the physician in a vignette described by Buckman told his leukemia patient what therapy he was recommending, he made sure she understood that they were battling a "very vicious illness," one that required strong treatment. Then he added about her chances:

> *"What we can't do at this time is absolutely guarantee that we can cure it forever for you, but there is a very high chance that we can squash it down flat and put you into remission with a few initial courses of strong drug therapy. That's what I think we can do."*

Similarly, when the general practitioner in Maguire's scenario told his patient that the cancer had returned (often the hardest news to give) and there was no purpose in treating it, he didn't promise that he could eliminate the pain. Instead, he said there was every chance that he could palliate it:

Doctor: "I'm sorry to have to tell you this. It can't be easy for you. Do you have any particular worries?"

Mr F: "I'm terrified of getting bad pain."

Doctor: "If that happens I hope we will be able to control your pain with strong painkillers. Let me know if you're having any problems with pain, or any other symptoms, come to that. The sooner we know about it the sooner we should be able to do something."

Even when the message was tough to tell, both physicians disposed of it without false assurance. Indeed, hope, especially when linked to treatment, is a necessary commodity, but only helpful when it's realistic. It does your patient little good if you say that you've seen 20 people respond to this treatment but fail to mention they're out of 20,000 cases. Also, while people identify the word *hope* with the word *cure*, it can have other meanings. Patients are hopeful, Baile suggests, if they hear about a therapy that's available despite the fact that it may not work. They're hopeful if they're receiving continuity of care and have access to expert opinions.

"The phrase, 'Fear the worst and hope for the best' has been around for a long time," says Baile. "But that's the kind of thing that we can offer our patients. We should be able to present the information without scaring the bejesus out of them. We should be helping patients accept reality and providing them with some level of hopefulness."

But in equipping them, you must also equip yourself. Quill already had sought out a close colleague with whom he could explore his own feelings of sadness before he dealt with those of his HIV patient. In so doing, he was able to quell many of her fears, and by the next visit she was fine and functioning.

> I think there's a mythology that if you just sit down and touch the patient and have tons of empathy it's going to make this harsh information inherently nonviolent. That's just not true. I was struggling to do the right thing with my patient, but my technique wasn't going to make it not devastating. The challenge is to really hang in there with the devastation, maintaining contact, and making sure that there's a plan.

Although it's been several years since Waldridge's first experience with breaking bad news—to that young man in a hospital bed—he's forever reminded of the lessons learned during that encounter: Organize the facts, engage the person, and show empathy.

Have his acquired skills made the process a walk in the park? Hardly, since each episode is still draining, and perfecting the process has become a lifelong pursuit. In the meantime, Waldridge takes solace in knowing that, as heart wrenching as breaking bad news can be, he may be doing it better than someone else might.

Finally, remember that while you're marshalling the coping mechanisms of your patients—and making sure they know you won't abandon them—they may be helping you in their own way. As Waldridge has experienced in some of the worst-case scenarios, "The biggest revelation has been how supportive my patients have been of *me*."

Bibliography

Brewin T. Three ways of giving bad news. *Lancet.* 1991;337:1207-1209.

Buckman R. *How to Break Bad News: A Guide for Health Care Professionals.* Baltimore, Md: Johns Hopkins University Press; 1992.

Cassem N, ed. The Dying Patient. In: *Massachusetts General Hospital Handbook of General Psychiatry.* 3rd ed. St Louis, Mo: Mosby Year Book; 1991.

Creagan E. How to break bad news—and not devastate the patient. *Mayo Clin Proc.* 1994;69:1015-1017.

Grigis A, Sanson-Fischer R. Breaking bad news: consensus guidelines for medical practitioners. *J Clin Oncol.* 1995;13:2449-2456.

Lind S, Good M, Seidel S, Csordas T, Good B. Telling the diagnosis of cancer. *J Clin Oncol.* 1989;7: 583-589.

Maguire P. Communicate with cancer patients: handling bad news and difficult questions. *Br Med J.* 1988;297:907-909.

Novack D, Plumer R, Smith R, Ochitill H, Morrow G, Bennett J. Changes in physicians' attitudes toward telling the cancer patient. *JAMA.* 1979;241:897-900.

Oken D. What to tell cancer patients: a study of medical attitudes. *JAMA.* 1961;175:1120-1128.

Quill T. Bad dews: delivery, dialogue, & dilemmas. *Arch Intern Med.* 1991;151:463-468.

Sardell A, Trierweiler S. Disclosing the cancer diagnosis. *Cancer.* 1993;72:3355-3365.

Waldridge R, Waldridge R II. Delivering bad news to patients and their families. *Fam Pract Manage 3.* 1996;No. 8:48-54.

Chapter 3

Cultural Competency: Turn Barriers into Bridges

Francesca Gany, MD, had a mystery on her hands. One by one, recent immigrants from the West African country of Senegal showed up at New York City's Bellevue Hospital with abdominal pains radiating around their waists to their backs. One by one, these men received extensive work-ups, upper GI series, barium enemas, ultrasounds, and stool studies. But as reliable as the clinical tests were, they didn't yield any clues. "Nobody," she says, "was getting anywhere."

Frustrated herself, Gany, who was in residency at the time, enlisted the aid of an anthropologist, who searched the local Senegalese community to find the missing puzzle piece. The abdominal pains were a manifestation of "toy," a somatization syndrome that is linked to stress due to overwork and the absence of family and friends.

At last, a diagnosis that made sense. Many of the men were new to this country, an ocean away from their rural roots and familial support. Many had never been to a Western physician and were seeking such help because they had no traditional healer in the city.

Once Gany and her colleagues knew the illness, they could address it. They matched the remedy normally prescribed, a gelatinous substance called "kell," in addition to "talk therapy." With Knox gelatin fortified by community support to relieve their patients' stress, Dr Gany and her colleagues devised an ingenious solution for a problem that didn't need high-tech biomedical help.

Not surprisingly, the men from Senegal improved. Gany, now executive director of the New York Task Force on Immigrant Health, achieved insight that has since influenced her practice. By going beyond the strictly clinical aspects of her medical training and exploring her patients' world, she could make a difference. As she observed:

> It was the first time I really delved into how someone's background could impact how they sought health care and the presentation of their symptoms, as well as how to work with patients to address those issues.

> I realized that to understand what's going on with the community as a whole, we have to take ourselves out of the medical setting and put ourselves into the patient's social setting or world to find out where this person is coming from in terms of their illnesses and health beliefs.

Practicing Medicine in a Melting Pot

As the country enters the next millennium, physicians such as Gany will have many opportunities to observe the culturally disparate worlds of their patients. By some accounts, 40% of the population in 2000 will be immigrants or first-generation Americans. By 2050, half are expected to be people of color.

These individuals represent a spectrum of populations from the smaller immigrations of Laotian peasant Hmong to the larger influx of Chinese, Japanese, and other sophisticated cultures whose philosophical, scientific, and medical traditions are well established, yet distinctly different from our own. Their presence means that more physicians will have to marshal communication and other skills to turn barriers into bridges across culture and language.

Like other aspects of medicine, interacting with people from all corners of the globe can be a complicated business even though the payoff is substantial: a deeper trust between yourself and your patient, not to mention improved compliance and outcomes. But such rewards occur only if you're aware of someone else's cultural beliefs, acknowledge that discrepancies exist between theirs and your own, and display an ability to meld the two. As M. Jean Gilbert, PhD, director of cultural competence for the California Division of Kaiser-Permanente, observes:

> What I always have to tell physicians is that the most important thing about culture is what's invisible—the norms, the values, the perspectives, the ideas. They're often not aware of those elements when a patient walks through the door. But it's those invisible aspects that are essential. Our challenge is in getting doctors to understand that differences among cultures are real and that they do affect the patient-healer relationship.

Becoming Culturally Competent

With a growing number of minorities finding their way into the American health system, fewer physicians will be able to ignore the special needs of a culturally diverse population: high rates of infectious disease, stress-related disorders tied to economic or cultural dislocations, and poor nutrition or other health problems linked to acculturation and a new environment.

Added to those concerns are the real differences between the medical beliefs or cultural practices of patients and their newfound providers. For distinctions exist on many fronts—from the way health care is accessed to the way it is delivered. In between are a number of variables that govern how patients view the anatomy, evaluate symptoms, treat or cure sickness, manage pain, and integrate traditional practices and healers with Western therapy and physicians.

Many people have explanatory models to describe the nature of illness—how it comes about, why it exists, and what can be done to prevent, control, or cure it. And frequently those notions differ from the biomedical model—a corpus of knowledge and style of discourse in which physicians are trained. But when physicians wear blinders or ignore the belief systems of their patients, they cannot be effective in identifying or treating their health care issues.

Of course, there's an alternative to this scenario, which is to provide what many health entities, including the American Medical Association (AMA), call "culturally competent health care," a catchphrase for a range of attributes, attitudes, behaviors, and policies that providers need to be effective in cross-cultural situations.

In its 1998 report, "Enhancing the Cultural Competence of Physicians," the AMA's Council on Medical Education describes physicians who provide this patient-centered care as "adjusting their attitudes and behaviors to the needs and desires of different patients and accounting for the impact of emotional, cultural, social, and psychological issues on the main biomedical ailment."

In personal terms, this means being aware of your own biases and mastering a set of tools (principally, interpersonal skills and the ability to implement what one group cited as a "trust-promoting method of inquiry") to work with people from differing populations.

Experts agree that culturally competent physicians recognize that every person's health beliefs are molded in large part by variables that may put a different emphasis on the role of religion, families, or even physicians. When those beliefs fall outside the realm of biomedicine (and inside the realm of "ethnomedicine"), these same physicians are willing to adapt their skills to accommodate those perspectives, even if they don't agree with the logic or efficacy. As Janet Madill, MD, medical director of the Legacy Clinic at Good Samaritan Hospital in Portland, Oregon, observes:

> I have a very strong sense that Western allopathic medicine, while it does many very good things, does not have all of the answers. So I try to approach each patient with a certain amount of humility and openness. I never see myself as an expert. I see myself as the constant learner.

Such openness, it could be argued, belongs at the heart of every encounter between patient and physician. Indeed it does. But conventional history-taking and physical examinations don't facilitate the kind of dialogue that fosters a *mutual* exchange of knowledge about health beliefs and practices. As J. Donald Mull, MD, MPH, writes in the November 1993 issue of *The Western Journal of Medicine*, current approaches are like an "algorithm designed to lead physicians to the single Oslerian diagnosis that explains all the symptoms."

Instead, physicians practicing across cultural barriers need to think like medical anthropologists to uncover the beliefs and behaviors of their patients. By becoming, as Mull suggests, a participant-observer in this individual's world, you're exploring like a scientist, alert to meanings your patient attaches to illness and sensitive to the social matrix that engulfs him or her. Both are crucial to your clinical success or failure, as is your ability to communicate in a culturally sensitive way.

Notice how switching gears made a difference for one medical student who had complained that she was learning nothing in her barrio clinic field project. People, she muttered to Mull, were answering her queries by asking, "How should I know why I'm sick? I've come to the doctor because he's the expert!"

But when he suggested that she change her approach—to talk first to patients about their lives and families—the folk beliefs began to flow. She learned, for example, that pregnant Mexican women wore bright new safety pins on their underwear to deflect dangerous rays from an eclipse, which they believed could cause a cleft lip in their babies.

This example underscores Mull's philosophy that medicine is really a "quintessential social science. To paraphrase what used to be said about anatomy, all physicians make mistakes, but those who know their anthropology make fewer of them."

Some Commonsense Tactics

A change of style on the physician's part may prompt a change of heart in the patient. But creating that milieu involves a number of commonsense tactics that can be summarized in any number of communication models.

For example, the mnemonic **LEARN** focuses physicians on how to elicit better patient acceptance by shifting the focus of their medical interviews from strict factual reports of symptoms to broader theoretical explanations of potential problems. Authors Elois Ann Berlin, PhD, and William C. Fowkes, MD, writing in the December 1983 issue of *The Journal of Western Medicine*, explain their framework this way:

"**L**" stands for "listen" with empathy to a patient's conceptualization of his or her illness;

"**E**" is to "explain" your own perceptions of the problem; "**A**" reminds you to

"acknowledge" the patient's explanatory model and to bridge any discrepancies between it and your own; "**R**" is for the treatment you "recommend" (including appropriate traditional remedies); and "**N**" stands for "negotiation" of a plan that reflects your decision-making partnership. (Emphasis added.)

Remember, the central issue in every cross-cultural clinical encounter is the transaction you have with your patient over your explanatory models. By evoking this person's views, you can learn a panoply of information: What beliefs does he or she hold about the illness, and which personal and social meanings does he or she attach to it? What are this person's expectations and therapeutic goals?

You may discover, for example, that your patient believes taking medicine over time weakens the blood. You then have to dispel the myth or suggest a tonic or vitamin in addition to the prescription. Or you may discover that when you use the words *high* and *low,* this individual thinks you're talking about blood sugar levels, when you're really referring to blood pressure.

In any case, the best way to learn is to ask, which requires thought and a systematic approach like the one suggested by Harvard University's Arthur Kleinman, MD, a medical anthropologist and one of the seminal thinkers in cross-cultural communication. Writing in the February 1978 issue of *Annals of Internal Medicine*, he constructed a set of simple and direct questions that are used widely to stimulate such discussion between physicians and patients.

You can learn, for example, which aspects of the clinical explanatory model you have to clarify and what patient education you'll need to pursue. You'll also be in a better position to address any conflicts that might surface in negotiating a therapeutic plan. To initiate your inquiry, Kleinman suggests asking your patient:

- What do you think has caused your problem?
- Why do you think it started when it did?
- What do you think your sickness does to you?
- How severe is your sickness?
- Will it have a short- or long-term course?
- What kind of treatment do you think you should receive?
- What are the most important results you hope to receive from this treatment?
- What are the chief problems your sickness has caused you?
- What do you fear most about your sickness?

You'll no doubt vary the wording to suit the person and his or her problem. But the key is to reach beyond the symptoms to the *perception* of this disease. Also, while direct questions may indeed reveal how one person views an illness, they may not work for everyone. In fact, you may find many patients who aren't forthcoming with their views—or worse, think you are uncertain about your own. This may call for you to alter your technique; suggest, for example, that you've heard similar comments from others in the community.

"We're trained to ask a lot of open-ended questions and that, to some patients, is very unnerving because they think that if you have to ask you really don't know what you're doing," Gany says. "So we have to work within those cultural beliefs to have credibility in the eyes of the patient."

When Lee M. Pachter, DO, associate professor of pediatrics and anthropology at the University of Connecticut School of Medicine, wanted to find out how the mother of Sammy, a 6-year-old asthmatic, was treating his respiratory attacks, he first asked her about prescriptions and over-the-counter medications. Then he paved the way for a discussion about folk remedy by saying:

> *"People have told me that there are ways to treat asthma that doctors don't know about. Usually they're recommended by grandparents and others who have had a lot of experience with the illness. Have you heard about any of these remedies?"*

By asking a general question, rather than appear to be prying, he took the onus out of the inquiry. Other indirect questions might be:

> *"What would an elder in your family say about this problem?"*
>
> *"What is this called in your language?"* or
>
> *"Patients who are ill the way you are tell me. . . ."*

Only when Sammy's mother affirmed that she *was* aware of folk remedies for treating asthma did Pachter follow up with a second series of questions:

> *"What are they?"*
>
> *"Are they effective?"*
>
> *"Have you ever tried (such and so) for your child's illness?"*
>
> *"Are you using it now?"*
>
> *"Is it helpful?"*

Pachter, who recounted his experience in the September 1997 issue of *Contemporary Pediatrics*, learned that when Sammy begins coughing and wheezing, his mother treats him with a syrup called *siete jarabes*, a folk remedy purchased at the local botanica. If Sammy doesn't get better within an hour, she follows with aerosol albuterol and, if that doesn't work, she then calls the physician.

Pachter first commended his patient for taking action. Then he told her that he didn't know if the *siete jarabes* would be effectual but he was satisfied that if it were given as directed, it wouldn't do any harm. Yet he also emphasized to her, "I am certain that the syrup would be much more effective if you follow it with an albuterol treatment right away, instead of waiting an hour."

By putting his patient's folk remedy in the context of the biomedical therapy he prescribed, he formed an alliance with the mother, creating a win-win situation. Indeed, since most medical beliefs don't interfere with biomedical treatment, you may be able to incorporate patients' individual therapies easily for illnesses that are mild or self-limiting.

Of course, you may need to take a harder stance if the cure is of questionable efficacy and expensive to boot. You may say to this patient, "If you're going to spend $800 for magnets to help your arthritis, I'd rather have you spend it on massage therapy." But nothing is lost if your patient wants to wear an amulet, burn incense, or consult a fortune-teller, so long as he or she still takes the penicillin you prescribe.

Likewise, the care you deliver won't be compromised if you invite a *santiguadora* or traditional healer into the hospital to help treat your Puerto Rican patient. You're simply being responsive to the concerns of the parents who are convinced that their child's *empacho*, a folk illness that's really a cultural gloss for gastroenteritis, will respond to her warm oil massage. In any case, just remember that you can't advise unless you know, and you can't know unless you ask, because your patients will probably not volunteer the information. As Melissa Welch, MD, MPH, chief medical officer at the Community Health Network of San Francisco, observes:

> Out of deference to you as a provider, most patients will not tell you the truth if you start to question or denigrate what they believe in. They'll just say, "Fine. I understand." But, in fact, they won't change what they're doing. So it's much better to acknowledge and try to partner with your patient rather than being very prescriptive.

Breaking Down Barriers

Your best intentions to be a partner, however, can go awry when belief systems are widely disparate and language barriers further complicate any efforts to span the gulf. In her book, *The Spirit Catches You and You Fall Down*, author Anne Fadiman provides a compelling picture of cultural miscommunication at its painful worst. Equally convinced about their interpretations of little Lia's seizures, her Merced, California, physicians clung fiercely to their Western beliefs that these episodes were caused by epilepsy, while her parents blamed them on *quag dab peg*, or "the spirit catches you and you fall down."

That was only the beginning. Plagued by a lack of suitable interpreters and a plethora of other problems, the physicians found their interactions with the family so intolerable that, at one point, they weren't sure if their inability to connect was due to cultural barriers or other, more insidious factors. The girl's pediatrician captures the frustration of this cultural gap:

> It felt as if there was this layer of Saran Wrap or something between us, and they were on one side of it and we were on the other side of it. And we were reaching and reaching and we could kind of get into their area, but we couldn't touch them. So we couldn't touch them. So we couldn't really accomplish what we were trying to do, which was to take care of Lia.

Indeed, lack of a common language (added to other factors) can be an impenetrable barrier. Yet even when you share a common culture and language with your patient, bear in mind that your specialized knowledge may seem to them as foreign as a second language.

But overcoming these gaps is crucial since complex issues underlie all patient-physician exchanges and language—carefully articulated and easily understood—is what drives your message home. When you can't communicate clearly or effectively, your ability to establish rapport, gather diagnostic information, and build a therapeutic alliance is impeded.

Also, some would suggest that a language barrier can prompt you to order unnecessary tests, interfere with your treatment plan, and even lead to worse outcomes. Several studies concerning asthmatics have shown, for example, that increased exacerbations and hospitalizations occur when there's no way to overcome language differences.

It would be wonderful if you could bridge the language barrier with your own linguistic dexterity. Indeed, greeting patients in their native tongue might be a great icebreaker. But with the profusion of languages, it's unrealistic to attempt to know each one. Gany, for instance, finds communicating in Spanish (in addition to French and a little of the West African language, Woulof) helpful in her practice. But she couldn't learn Mandarin quickly enough to communicate effectively with the increasing number of Chinese patients she sees who speak it.

A little fluency might put you in good stead with the elder of the family. Yet when the discussion turns to serious medical issues, the communication task becomes trickier. Ideally, you may want to enlist the aid of a professional interpreter, schooled in the terminology of medicine, rather than a staff person or your patient's next of kin.

Family members are not necessarily the wisest choice, even though they are sometimes the only ones available. They usually don't understand biomedical concepts or medical terminology. They're less likely to understand why you're asking certain questions and more likely to filter their responses in an effort to please you. In addition, they then become privy to your patient's confidential health information.

Further, while someone's next of kin may hold the key to important medical and family history, this person also may have an agenda that gets in the way of your patient's welfare. You're not likely to learn from an abusive husband, for example, that the bruises on his wife were inflicted by him.

Obviously, not all family relations are nefarious. An adult son or daughter may simply be overprotective of his or her parents or put off by their practices. Family members often "edit and polish," says Gany, to hide their embarrassment over old-world beliefs. They may not reveal, for example, that their Chinese grandfather is eating crocodile soup for his sadness or that their grandmother is seeing the herbalist for her many maladies.

In addition, family members often lose their objectivity and neutrality. Using a young girl's uncle as an interpreter, Pachter had him ask the Southeast Asian parents if they wanted to withdraw life support from their brain-dead daughter. The uncle reported back to Pachter that they weren't ready to take that step. But the reality of the girl's situation was never relayed to her mother and father. The uncle just couldn't tell his brother that the girl was dying.

This story is a poignant example of the need to be judicious when using relatives as translators, even adults. Obviously, in some situations you may not have a choice; and your predicament may be further complicated if you have to rely on a child or adolescent. For example, the only person to speak for a 12-year-old patient may be his or her 15-year-old brother. Or you may be facing a life-and-death situation in the ER and have to explain the options to a teenage son or daughter. But the fact remains: Most youngsters cannot advance the conversation because they lack familiarity with medical nuances and jargon. And nobody wants to subject a child to undue trauma.

In fact, if your interpretation needs overwhelm a relative, you may be the unwitting source of family stress. In many cultures, it's disrespectful to place a young person in a position of power over an elder, even though it may be inevitable given the English proficiency of second-generation Americans. But calling on them to interpret can lead, as Gany asserts, "to really bad psychosocial issues within the family."

Similarly, assigning the task to one of your own employees interrupts the work flow, slows operations, and can result in resentment on the part of coworkers. Moreover, even though nurses are trained in the nuances of complex medical material and know to keep confidences, they may not have a command of the target language. Or they could be influenced by their own biases and resist being associated with your patient's beliefs.

Robert W. Putsch III, MD, writing in the December 20, 1985, issue of the *Journal of the American Medical Association*, describes how one Spanish-American head nurse consistently withheld information about folk therapies:

> Patients shouldn't believe those things. I tell them that and I don't translate what they say to the doctors. . . . I don't think we should discuss things like that in a place like this—it makes it look like we approve of it. . . . What with my position here and all, it doesn't seem right to talk about it. This place is dedicated to modern medicine. . . . If I tell the doctors, they might think that I believe in that too.

With a little in-service education, this nurse understood how someone's practices might play a role in therapy and eventually provided highly educational commentary. But her initial attitude points out the importance of tapping people for this task who are able to deal honestly and openly with issues that have heavy cultural overtones.

In fact, if you're a monolingual physician interacting with a monolingual patient, your ideal option is to hire a trained medical interpreter who is fully conversant in the concepts, terminology, and procedures of biomedicine and also knowledgeable about this individual's culture. This professional has sufficient experience in patient encounters and the intricacies of interpreted communication to be able to link information efficiently and effectively between the two of you.

Although nothing can replace the immediacy of a direct connection, if you're fortunate enough to have an expert interpreter who is also a good interviewer, then language barriers may be less of an issue.

Also, good medical interpreters can serve as "cultural consultants" for all parties. They improve continuity when many practitioners are involved. They expedite access to care by explaining patient rights and the mechanics of the health system. Finally, they facilitate trust between individuals, their families or community, and the health care providers or programs.

The downside is that trained medical interpreters can be expensive, especially if your practice is small and your patients come from many parts of the world. A second option is a telephone translation service such as the AT&T Language Line, which links physicians with bilingual interpreters who are available seven days a week. Often native speakers, they're prescreened and undergo special training. However, telephone translation *is* impersonal. The interpreters may not know the local dialects or slang of the patient with whom you're dealing, and it's impossible for a phone translator to assess nonverbal cues.

At Madill's clinic, paid professional medical interpreters are the communication conduit physicians use to talk with patients whose native tongues are as disparate as Russian and Chinese, Thai and Spanish. They usually have a good grasp of how to convey the medical situation in the language being interpreted. This creates what she calls a communication "triad," in which everyone is contributing something valuable. "I find it helpful when medical interpreters are willing to not only translate what's going on, but to act as cultural brokers," she says. "I try to let them know that I'm open to more than just the literal translation."

Is there room for miscommunication? Of course. Confusion can happen any time two people exchange information. But Madill's approach is to be open to learning at every juncture and to ask more questions when things "don't feel quite right."

In fact medical interpreting can be fraught with problems, no matter who does the translating. While the head nurse in Putsch's example was worried about her self-image, other trained interpreters can have similar problems. Even when an interpreter is from the same culture, he or she may have difficulty melding certain differences, such as those that may occur if the translator and patient are from different socioeconomic backgrounds—urban versus rural for example.

Indeed, by introducing a third party into the conversation, you're adding another human being who is subject to his or her own foibles and fears. Madill recalls the female interpreter who ran out of the room when Madill started a full exam of her male Russian patient. The patient found it amusing, but it was clear that the translator was too embarrassed to continue translating.

While it may seem awkward to invite an interpreter into the examination room, one should be present if possible, even if he or she stands behind a curtain, says Gany. After all, if you were the patient, would you want to be probed without understanding what the doctor was doing?

Granted, the time constraints of managed care render it difficult to have tête-à-têtes with the translator prior to the patient encounter. But by consulting together beforehand, you can outline your goals, discuss problems such as medication compliance, and possibly learn from the translator those cultural differences that affect patient care.

You may learn, for example, that when your Native American patient stares at the floor, it's not out of defiance. Rather, diverting one's eyes is a show of respect. Or you'll know to avoid contact with the left hand of a Middle Eastern immigrant because that's the hand they use for such things as blowing their nose.

At any rate, a preliminary discussion with the interpreter is an opportune time to let him or her know you want a word-for-word translation. That way you're more likely to get the nuances of a literal interpretation. Moreover, you should emphasize that even if the patient's answer doesn't pertain directly to your question—or even borders on the superstitious—you want to hear it.

At the same time, make sure your interpreter is aware that careless phrasing and omissions can change meanings. Miscommunication occurs when messages are paraphrased or two separate and unrelated issues are mingled. A carefully worded statement might end up as a roughly approximated version. Or an interpreter's minor omission may result in a crucial missed comment.

The following exchange, cited initially by British surgeon John Launer, MA, MB, in the September 30, 1978, *British Medical Journal*, exemplifies what can happen between physicians and their Nigerian patients when the conversation is filtered through medical orderlies:

> *Patient (in Hausa):* "It's my ear that's hurting me. It's blocked and I can't hear with it. The head and neck are hurting and I've got a fever."
>
> *Interpreter:* "She says she's suffering from ear pain and headache."
>
> Or
>
> *Patient (in Hausa):* "This leg. There's pain inside it in the night. In the afternoon I can't walk around freely. If I bend it, I can't straighten it due to the pain."
>
> *Interpreter:* "He has pain in the right leg. Right inside the bone."

Also, while physicians traditionally have used a "triadic," or triangular, configuration to facilitate communication, an interpreter can be seated next to you with your patient directly across from you both. If facing two professionals is too threatening for the patient, then seat yourself opposite both of them or place the interpreter slightly behind, but within earshot, of your patient, yet also within your sight. Gany and her colleagues even advise interpreters to look down, or even close their eyes, to seem less of an intrusion to the patient.

No matter how you position everyone, the exchange is always between physician and patient, even though the interpreter must be involved. If a staff member translates, make sure he or she isn't engaged in any other tasks simultaneously. The physician also should not divert his or her attention from the patient's nonverbal clues—facial expressions, body language, and length of responses.

Once situated, the process for an effective encounter is fairly straightforward: Speak in short sentences so the translator can easily follow your train of thought. Drop the medical jargon and avoid colloquialisms, abstractions, idioms, slang, similes, and metaphors (eg, words like *work-up* should be conveyed in plain English). Avoid terms such as *would, could, if,* and *maybe.* Their ambiguity can be confusing to a foreign-speaking person.

Instead, Putsch suggests that physicians phrase things so an interpreter can translate easily and "break down" information when a lengthy explanation is needed. Also, make allowances for terms that don't exist in your patient's language. This vignette from Putsch's *JAMA* article is a good example.

> *Physician:* "Would you ask her if she is allergic to any medications?"
>
> *Navajo Interpreter:* "Does the white man's medicine make you vomit?"
>
> *Patient:* "No."
>
> *Physician:* "That's not quite what I need to know. I have to know about allergies to medications."
>
> *Interpreter:* "Well, I don't know about those things. What's 'allergy' mean anyway?"

Like such terms as *anxiety* and *depression, bacteria* and *diabetes, allergy* is a biomedical abstraction, writes Putsch, that has no concept among certain cultures. But such concepts need not escape translation. Putsch suggests an alternative to the above scenario that would likely yield a trove of information, even if the medical concept is a mystery to that culture:

> *"Did you ever have a rash from a medication? Did you ever have breathing troubles from a medication? {and the like}"*

By eliciting specific, rather than vague, responses, you can better deduce symptoms and determine an accurate diagnosis. Invite specific information with statements such as "Correct me if I'm wrong, but I understood it this way." Or pursue seemingly unconnected issues. This may lead to critical information.

Among your list of do's and don'ts, *do* repeat information, especially when it involves treatment. Then go one step further and ask your patient to repeat it back to you. *Don't* hesitate to interrupt the interview to seek clarification. *Do* ask the interpreter to convey the entire conversation if it has gone beyond a simple yes or no response.

Finally, remember that what's familiar to you may not be to someone else. David Waters, MD, a pediatrician at Milwaukee's 16th Street Community Health Center, which serves one of the city's many multicultural neighborhoods, recalls a Hmong child whose meningitis led to hydrocephalus, which necessitated a ventriculo-peritoneal shunt.

The parents, keeping vigil at their daughter's hospital bedside, were hesitant about the procedure. (Hmong, in general, are wary of surgery because they're afraid the doctor might remove an organ they believe must be with them when they die.) So the neurosurgeon—a "delightfully caring individual"—used a popular American sports image to describe what would happen to the little girl's head if he didn't insert the shunt. But his analogy didn't score many points. The child's parents looked quizzically at the interpreter and asked, "What's a basketball?" "He was trying to make this dramatic point to them but it was completely lost," says Waters. "It wasn't anything in their experience."

Hitting a Home Run

Perhaps you've been stymied by a predicament similar to that described above. The comparisons you draw or the point you want to drive home falls short. As the neurosurgeon discovered, good intentions and great similes often aren't enough to communicate successfully with patients from different cultures. These acts must be reinforced by those essential attributes—rapport, empathy, support, partnership, and trust.

Yet none of these communication skills, say physicians, are ever really perfected and certainly aren't mastered overnight. With today's time constraints limiting patient encounters to as few as 10 or 12 minutes, it's hard to build rapport in one visit. You need to somehow demonstrate that you're in it for the long haul. Further, physicians are most effective when they incorporate these communication skills into their own individual style, determined by what's comfortable and what works.

Welch has a personal goal in mind when she starts up a conversation with any of the ethnically diverse patients she sees through San Francisco's county health care delivery system. Before launching into her medical agenda, the physician looks for some commonality—perhaps she's visited the patient's homeland—that could foster a personal connection. Taking this step, says Welch, reminds the patient of his or her individuality. From there, her emphasis shifts to this triad: be aware of this patient's unique culture; assess and treat him or her in light of their practices; and don't make any assumptions about his or her beliefs.

It's this last point that may be the most important one for every physician working through the complexities of a cross-cultural encounter: never assume anything. For there is heterogeneity to all cultures. Individual differences in terms of health knowledge—as well as attitude and behavior—within ethnic communities are significant, often influenced by education, social class, and even acculturation.

Also, patient beliefs are often not what appearances may suggest. People meet Welch, for example, and assume by the color of her skin that she's African-American when, in fact, her heritage is a blend of Latin American and Caribbean. Born in Panama, she spoke Spanish before English, and her belief systems center around those cultures. This has taught Welch to test her own assumptions.

Which brings us back to the lessons learned from Gany's experience with her Senegalese patients. An anthropologist may help you figure out what's going on with an entire population. But the best way to learn about a single patient is to focus on that person and encourage him or her to *lead you*. As Gany notes:

> We have to let every patient be his or her own medical anthropologist. We all have our own "culture" within our greater culture so we never can assume that generalities apply to the individual we're seeing. When we're in the room with this patient, we have to put the larger cultural norms in the background and go to this person for the specifics. We just need to let our patients be our guide.

Bibliography

Berlin E, Fowkes W. A teaching framework for cross-cultural health care. *West J Med*. 1983;139:934-938.

Buchwald D, Caralis P, Gany F, Hardt E, Muecke M, Putsch R. The medical interview across cultures. *Patient Care*. April 15, 1993:142-166.

Clark M. Cultural context of medical practice. *West J Med*. 1983;139:806-810.

Fadiman A. *The Spirit Catches You and You Fall Down: A Hmong Child, Her American Doctors and the Collision of Two Cultures*. New York, NY: Farrar, Strauss & Giroux; 1997.

Kaufert J, Putsch R. Communication through interpreters in healthcare: ethical dilemmas arising from differences in class, culture, language and power. *J Clin Ethics*. 1997;8:71-87.

Kleinman A. Culture, illness and care: clinical lessons from anthropologic and cross-cultural research. *Ann Intern Med*. 1978;88:251-258.

Kraut A. Healers and strangers: immigrant attitudes toward the physician in America—a relationship in historical perspective. *JAMA*. 1990;263:1807-1811.

Lieberman L, Stoller E, Burg M. Women's health care: cross-cultural encounters within the medical system. *J Fla Med Assoc*. 1997;84:364-373.

Mull J. Cross-cultural communication in the physician's office. *West J Med*. 1993;159:609-613.

Pachter L. Culture and clinical care: folk illness beliefs and behaviors and their implications for health care delivery. *JAMA*. 1994;271:690-694.

Pachter L. Practicing culturally sensitive pediatrics. *Contemp Pediatr 14*. 1997;No. 9:139-154.

Putsch R. Cross-cultural communication: the special case of interpreters in health care. *JAMA*. 1985;254:3344-3348.

Putsch R, Joyce M. Dealing with patients from other cultures. In: *Clinical Methods*. 3rd ed. Boston, Mass: Butterworths; 1990:1050-1065.

Waters D. Providing health care for the Hmong. *Wis Med J*. 1992;91:642-651.

Welch M. Cross-cultural communication. In Feldman MD, Christensen JF, eds. *Behavioral Medicine in Primary Care: A Practical Guide*. Stamford, Conn: Appleton & Lange; 1997:97-108.

Chapter 4

The Role of the Family: No Patient Is an Island

Isaac Bloch's baby-sitter knew the drill. When an X-acto knife accidentally penetrated the 6-year-old's right eye, she rushed to notify his physician as well as family. Within 30 minutes, the two of them were in the Manhattan Eye and Ear Hospital, where physicians worked feverishly to repair Isaac's eye. Outside the operating room, the boy's paternal grandfather (himself a physician) and maternal grandmother had arrived in lieu of his parents to sign the necessary papers for surgery. Because the grandparents promptly stepped in for Isaac's parents, who were not immediately available, the physicians could perform their miracles. Isaac was in good hands. He eventually regained 20/40 vision in that eye.

There's a lesson to be learned for all health care professionals from medical crises such as this: Families are the health care resource of both first and last resort. Granted, physicians have the expertise and proficiency, but it's the family that plays a continuing role in a patient's medical condition. Says Isaac's grandfather, Donald A. Bloch, MD, who is cochairman of the Collaborative Family Healthcare Coalition:

> Isaac's grandmother and I were able to make a difference. We could get important emergency care underway quickly. But many times families have to hang in there with a child who's getting chemotherapy for cancer or a spouse who's battling a chronic illness like diabetes. The doctor sets up the regimen. Maybe the visiting nurse comes in to help. But the family is there 24 hours a day.

Pain in the Neck or Positive Force?

Developing trust with the families of your patients may be your most critical communication challenge. Getting a pulse, figuratively speaking, on those who know your patient best can help you get a pulse on the patient. It also can produce a trove of information that will help *you* help your patient.

Granted, in an emergency such as Isaac's, physicians need to move quickly. But more often than not, time will be on your side. Over months, if not years, you'll have many opportunities to get a sense of a patient's family life. Through both direct questions and astute observations, you can piece together their unique dynamics. Unfortunately, physicians often underestimate the influence of family on their patient and fail to enlist them as a resource. Instead, they may interact with the family in a perfunctory way—as people entitled to hear the results of surgery or a physical—but not much more.

Blame it on a culture that treasures autonomy, but families are rarely viewed as active partners in the medical care of individual patients. We could learn much from other cultures, where families play such an important role that you may find yourself dealing with the group elder instead of directly with the patient. Granted, certain specialties—such as family medicine and pediatrics—put a premium on "family-oriented" medicine, which places the patient in a larger context. In such practices, physicians try to understand their patient's personal relationships and emotional ties with extended family, as well as cross-generational patterns.

But in most specialties, physicians aren't taught such skills, even though virtually every practice of medicine may eventually involve them. The sad result is that many even have difficulty expressing the basics to families. Whether you're the oncologist delivering news of cancer or the neurologist confirming a brain disorder, you may deliver the diagnosis to the patient, but this information resonates beyond him or her. Whether you're an orthopedic surgeon discussing hip surgery or a gasteroenterologist talking about colon tumors, you may hear from family members who call with questions and concerns.

Remember, it's family members who often fill in the blanks about your patient's health history. It's family members who correct misconceptions and catch the nuances of what you're saying. And it's family members who are there emotionally and even physically for individual patients. Case Western Reserve University researchers Jack H. Medalie, MD, MPH, and his colleagues note that in 32% of all family practice office visits, family members were present. The results of their study, published in the May 1998 issue of *The Journal of Family Practice*, also reports that in 18% of those visits, another family member's problems were discussed and 10% of the time was devoted to family issues.

"Family members are working on the same issues that you are, whether you're aware of it or not," says Steven R. Hahn, MD, associate professor of medicine and instructor in psychiatry, Albert Einstein College of Medicine of Yeshiva University. "Obviously you want them to work with you. You want to empower them to be your assistant. That's extremely important because the chronic illnesses that we deal with often cause dysfunction and require tremendous amounts of self-care. Patients need a lot of compensatory support from family members and you want to enlist them in giving it."

Defining the "Family"

Most of us define "family" based on our own personal experience. Maybe ours was the image Norman Rockwell put to canvas in the 1950s. But today the canvas is one of many images. It could be a single parent with children or cohabiting couples with none. Foster-parent households or divorcees blending their clans through second marriages. Gay relationships or adopted families. People who define kinship in terms of friends from work or who they know through church and synagogue. They all make up the portrait we call the American family today.

What *hasn't* changed, however, is that most people still get their physical and emotional needs met through family—whatever form that takes. Regardless of what we perceive to be family, it's within this context that most of us develop our beliefs, including our views on health.

"The family is the matrix of identity," says Alexander Blount, EdD, associate professor and director of behavioral science in family medicine and community health at the University of Massachusetts, Worcester. "It's how people develop their sense of who they are physically, as well as who they are in terms of personality type or style.

"There are families in which small pains are big tragedies and need to be worried about. {Then there} are families in which small pains are signs of weakness and should never be shown. All of the training about who we are and how we are in our bodies is developed in the family."

There's also a powerful body of scientific evidence that suggests that family members influence each other's health status. In the book *Family-Oriented Primary Care* that he coauthored, Thomas L. Campbell, MD, outlines three areas that seem to be affected: family stress on illness, family lifestyles on cardiovascular risks, and family function on chronic disease.

Since 1967 the Social Readjustment Rating Scale by Holmes and Rahe has provided subjective ratings for 43 of life's most stressful events. With death of a spouse leading the list, many of the other episodes—eg, divorce, personal injury or illness, and pregnancy—involve the family. The Holmes-Rahe scale has led to numerous studies showing that the incidence of both serious and minor illness, such as childhood asthma and respiratory ailments, can increase with stress.

Similarly, there's evidence to suggest that family members share the same lifestyle patterns and risk factors for coronary artery disease. The Framingham Heart Study, for instance, established parallels between spouses in their blood pressure and blood sugar, cholesterol, and triglyceride levels. Additionally, individuals find it more or less difficult to change their bad habits if they're shared with other family members.

Smokers, for example, are more likely to stop for good if no one else close to them smokes or if their spouses support them.

Further, several chronic illnesses depend on the involvement of others for good outcomes. Dysfunctional families (absent fathers, poor living conditions, chronic conflict, and lack of parental involvement with the disease) often cause poor control of diabetes, for example. Conversely, good family organization, high parental self-esteem, and emotional closeness can improve it. All of this is to say that families can be the conduit for information your patient may have difficulty sharing with you, as well as a tool you can use to increase cooperation and explain complicated medical regimens.

"I always look at the family as a source for helping us make progress," says Julie Dostal, MD, associate program director, department of family practice, Lehigh Valley Hospital, Allentown, Pennsylvania. "In difficult times, they can be a support and ally in moving things along and finding ways to make things work."

Finding an Opening

How much you learn about a patient's family—and when you learn it—often depends on your own goals with that patient. Very often you can't miss the family dynamic because members will invariably interact with you through questions and concerns. Or perhaps your patient will innocuously suggest something is awry at home. He or she may complain of general uneasiness or have aches and pains that appear so psychosomatic they beg the question, "How are things going?"

In any case, there are tools to help you identify the players in every family's drama. A genogram, for example, effectively summarizes the history and relationships of a patient's family while it pinpoints the forces at play. Genograms are used by family therapists to analyze "family systems." This theoretical lens can help physicians practice family-oriented care. The genogram builds on the standard medical history by collecting useful information about a patient's family. It allows physicians quick access to complex information about both physical and psychological health patterns. Because it's a chart, a physician can analyze the material quickly, noting how certain family members might react to a crisis by being either a source of support or a cause of stress.

Campbell, for instance, could identify potential family problems with a lung cancer patient whose children, except for one son, seemed unable to provide for her care. The genogram showed him that her other son had mild retardation and her daughter—who had been sexually abused by the patient's boyfriend—was unwilling to see her mother while he was still around. The information contained in the genogram made it clearer who could be there for this patient and what issues might surface as her terminal illness progressed. "It's the difference," he says, "between really getting to know the patient as a person versus just getting to know him or her as someone who might have a disease."

The beauty of genograms is that they're acceptable to patients and relatively simple, especially if you focus on core family members and current issues. (A comprehensive, or expanded, genogram goes beyond the nuclear family to encompass generations.) Their schematic consists of single lines that link spouses and outline households; double lines that indicate strong bonds; triple lines to depict close connections that are dysfunctional; and dotted or jagged lines that mark conflicted relationships.

What's included depends entirely on the patient's condition and the degree to which their family situation might affect care. Starting with baseline data (such as age and cause of death of other family members), a genogram also may include such important life events as marriage or divorce, as well as any major illnesses. From there, the more you ask, the more you learn. Although a genogram is not hard to master, it may feel like an added burden at first. Yet physicians who've used them in their practice say the payoff can be enormous, especially in unmasking "difficult" patients and family dysfunction. If your patient is healthy enough, expanded genograms aren't necessary. But with those whose health problems are acute or chronic, the more you know about their family life the better. The good news is that because genograms are databases, they can be revised as a situation changes. Also, they trigger a closer examination of a family's transitional stages. Every cycle— newlywed, raising children, or nearing retirement and old age—presents its own challenges or stresses that may affect your patient's health.

By searching the genogram, family therapist Joanne Cohen, PhD, discovered the underlying cause for a toddler's drastic weight gain. His parents, a young African-American couple, were referred to Cohen (who works in collaboration with Dostal) when physicians couldn't find an organic reason for the increased weight. Cohen learned that the boy's mother, who was 18, had left her home in the South 2 years earlier to marry the baby's father. They then lived near her husband's family and his mother was overfeeding the boy.

Once Cohen recognized the pattern, she was able to work with the young couple and get the husband to support his wife by drawing boundaries around their family unit. She also encouraged him to talk to his mother about how he and his wife wanted the baby fed. Soon after, the child began to lose weight and the young mother felt more in control as a parent. "This was a young family attempting to differentiate from their own families of origin," Cohen says. "And that's always a point of real transition and stress. It's also a potential time for intervention."

Granted, not all cases require direct intervention. However, in *Behavioral Medicine in Primary Care*, Hahn suggests that by asking a series of open-ended questions, you can discover how the family functions overall, as well as what may directly affect your patient. Even if you suspect a source of stress, it's important not to make any assumptions and to begin generally. For example,

> *"I know that all families have their ups and downs. How is yours doing these days with all that is going on in your life?"*

From there you can progress to more specific questions, such as, "Are you having problems with (your spouse, child, sibling, parent)?" Or shift the focus to your patient's condition: "How is your family dealing with your diabetes?" You can vary the approach to glean more details by asking how a particular family member is reacting to the patient's illness, for example. In short, you can vary your approach to suit the circumstances.

Perhaps you suspect dysfunction in the family, given clues you're getting from the patient. He isn't complying with treatment and instead continues to binge or smoke. She complains about mood swings and other more diffuse symptoms. They've been into your office time and again, yet resist your counsel and advice. Whether it be depression or domestic violence, divorce or death, any number of factors can lead to family dysfunction. Whatever the predicament, Hahn suggests you ask questions that will reveal how the patient and his or her family is adapting. For example:

> *"I know you have been feeling quite depressed lately; how has your family reacted to that?"*
> or

> *"What does your family think about the suggestions I've made?"*

Usually such exchanges will provide a springboard for subsequent discussion or interventions. Being open and up-front with family members not only enhances an alliance over your patient's medical condition, it also helps you better manage the condition. "As physicians we need to be aware that our patients have families," says Campbell. "We need to get them included in the discussions. Unfortunately, our culture tends to be so individually focused that in medicine the emphasis is often on protecting the patient from the family. The family is seen as intrusive—as opposed to concerned and supportive—which is the way most patients view it."

Reliable Sources

The communication skills you use with family members are the same ones that apply to patients. Build rapport. Gather information. Then educate, negotiate, and motivate. Once you add more people to the mix, you also add more complexities to the exchange. Every voice needs to be heard, and you are the one to orchestrate it all. How you perform this task can foster a patient's well-being and a family's cooperation.

A number of misconceptions and missteps on the part of physicians can impede helpful family involvement. For instance, they may assume that the trusting relationship they've built with the individual patient extends to the patient's family. Or they may overlook the fact that, although they have their patient's attention in the office, others have it at home. Sometimes physicians treat family members with benign neglect. At best, they may view them as idle spectators. At worst, they may think of them as an intrusion. "Instead," says Campbell, "the goal should be to say, 'We're interested in you and your opinion about how your loved one is doing.' We should be helping them feel like valued members of the healthcare team."

There are many points at which involving family members is appropriate, if not necessary. But the first step is to ask your patient for permission. In this way you're respecting the trust the two of you have built, as well as reassuring your patient you'll stay mindful of him or her during the conversation. Obtaining permission can be approached a number of ways:

> *"I think it would really be helpful for you to bring your daughter along next time so we could talk about your treatment."*

> *"Would you mind if we ask your husband to come in before you leave today so we could discuss these dietary changes?"* or

> *"Hello, I'm Dr So-and-So. I don't think we've met. And who are you?"* (Then to your patient): *"Would you like your son to stay here while we chat?"*

By taking a few minutes to find what Campbell calls a "common language," you're making the family member feel part of the conversation. In short, take time for some small talk. The point is to show your enthusiasm for the family member's participation. Once you've dispensed with the preliminaries, you then can delve into the matter at hand:

> *"How do you think your dad's been doing since his surgery?"*

> *"I'd like your perspective on how your mom is managing her blood sugar."* or

> *"Do you have any questions about your son's progress?"*

Once you've made the human connection, you've paved the way for any important explanations, observations, or concerns that a family member can offer. You might discover from a relative, for example, that the colon cancer your patient says her mother died from was actually liver disease. Or it might be something less tangible, but equally crucial to an accurate diagnosis. Hepworth tells the story of a young boy who had trouble getting up for school each morning in the fall because of stomach pains. By probing into the family history, the physician learned that when the mother was herself a teen, her father died from a lingering illness in the autumn. Now, as her son approached the age she'd been at the time of her loss, she became more and more depressed when autumn arrived. As the present caught up with her past, she was reminded of how hard it had been for her to leave for school because of anxiety that her father might die while she was gone. Her son, picking up on her uneasiness, simply manifested the symptoms. By bringing what was unconscious to the surface, the physician helped the mother lessen her son's apprehension. He encouraged her to be upbeat about sending her son off to school, which in turn was easier for her once she was assured the boy's stomach aches weren't serious.

This vignette exemplifies how forging an alliance between patient and family can net positive results. To get there, however, you have to deal with existing coalitions in all their permutations. You may need to reassure family members that each of their viewpoints is important in finding solutions. In his book, Campbell tells of the parents of a diabetic boy who began their conversation with the physician by blaming each other for inappropriate care of their son's illness. The mother wasn't giving him the right foods, according to the father. The father wasn't home enough to know what the boy ate, said the mother. The physician nipped the problem in the bud by saying:

> *"It's clear you both have a perspective that will be important to hear. You both are obviously concerned about your son or you wouldn't be here today. Let's begin with Ralph [the son] and hear what problems he feels he's having sticking to his diet."*

By maintaining his neutrality, this physician provided necessary leadership and steered the conversation in a productive direction. But the aim of your comments and questions is to further your health care goals and to clarify each individual's involvement. Give everyone the chance to speak, even if you have to draw them into the conversation. If someone is sitting off to the side, for example, let him or her know that you want to hear their opinion. You could say,

> *"Since we've just met, Mrs Smith, I'd like your perspective on your dad's progress. Perhaps you could sit closer to us so I can hear you."* or

> *"Mrs Smith, why don't you move your chair closer to us so I have everyone in my range of vision. Good. Can you tell me how your dad was responding before you brought him to the emergency room?"*

Hearing everyone's point of view also means making sure no one dominates the conversation. This is one approach:

> *"Ms Power, I'd like to hear more from you, but first I want to get your sister's viewpoint about your mom's condition. Then, if we have time, we'll come back to you."*

Yet the more people there are in the conversation, the more variability there will be among their medical knowledge and expectations. Ask each one how he or she perceives the problem and acknowledge the accuracy to determine what information should follow. Research has shown that families influence each other's lifestyle choices and modify behavior. You'll increase cooperation by identifying those closest to your patient. Spouses, for example, are often key to ensuring that your patient follows an exercise program or takes his or her medication.

When the patient in a vignette suggested by Campbell said she knew she needed to reduce her meal portions and avoid sweets to control her diabetes, her husband wanted to know if that meant the whole family had to change diets. The physician's response was, "How do you feel about that?" When the husband said he felt he should support his wife, but was worried he would resent giving up some foods, the physician replied:

> *"Many aspects of your wife's diet are part of good nutrition, so you may want to use this as an opportunity to change some of your family's eating habits. But it is very important that family members not sacrifice too much or resentments will build. You and your wife can be creative and find alternative foods for her to eat when the rest of the family wants dessert."*

The husband responded, "I understand. We will work on this together. Her well-being is important to all of us."

Calling All Relatives

Many times, the information you need to share with families can be provided informally in your office. Yet there are times when scheduled family conferences are the best approach. They're essential when you need immediate, direct intervention for specific issues, such as noncompliance and unexpected illnesses. Other obvious moments are when your patient is in a transition or the situation seems intractable. Emotions may be running high, and you can't see making progress without assembling the family. But there are other times—markers if you will—when calling a family meeting is the rule rather than the exception. Campbell suggests them for the following situations:

- **Hospitalizations.** Whether the admission is because of an acute event, such as myocardial infarction; a chronic illness such as asthma; or the end-stage of a terminal illness, a family meeting can further understanding about treatment and prognosis.

- **Death and dying.** Whether family members are hearing a diagnosis of terminal illness or learning of a death, a meeting can help them deal with their shock and grief.

- **Diagnosis of a serious chronic illness.** Whether it's diabetes or heart disease, bringing family members together may help you identify the best support for your patient.

- **Routine pregnancy and well-child care.** Encouraging formal meetings with fathers or significant others is an important step in reinforcing their parenting roles. Campbell insists, for example, that soon-to-be dads attend at least one prenatal appointment during each half of the pregnancy, along with a well-child visit within the first 6 months after the birth.

You may become so adroit at handling these formal sessions that you choose to schedule them routinely with all new patients. By bringing the family together at the outset, you show how much you value their involvement. In any event, when requesting a meeting you want to be positive and direct, emphasizing that it's routine in a case like this or that you find it useful to involve family members. Focus on the importance of the family, noting that it's helpful to get additional perspectives. Always acknowledge that the patient's condition might cause others pain and that perhaps everyone will benefit from the meeting.

Response from family members may very well be positive. In a study published in the November 5, 1986, issue of *The Journal of Family Practice*, Kenneth Kushner, PhD, and his colleagues reported that 30% of study participants had experienced family meetings and many were greatly satisfied. While the participants reported a moderate to low interest in having such conferences for minor issues, they expressed a high interest in them for serious ones. However, not every patient will be keen about meeting with parents, siblings, or significant others, especially if there's already strife. You'll want to be alert to any undertones when you approach your patient on the subject of their family.

Jeri Hepworth, PhD, professor, department of family medicine, and associate residency director, The University of Connecticut School of Medicine, and St Francis Hospital and Medical Center, Hartford, wishes she had paid closer attention when a newly diagnosed AIDS patient warned her and her colleagues that telling his parents—with whom he lived—would only wreak havoc. They would not only hate hearing the diagnosis, he predicted, but the exchange would be "just awful." Optimistic, Hepworth kept saying, "Oh, no. We'll just bring them in and of course they'll understand. They always do."

But just as the young man warned, the scene was dreadful. The mother, in particular, wouldn't focus on her son's illness. She simply couldn't get past the lifestyle that had resulted in his AIDS. Luckily, Hepworth and her physician-colleague could handle the vitriol that ensued. But ideally, she admits, had they paid more attention to the patient's words, they might have met with the mother separately first so she could vent her nasty rhetoric on them, rather than on her dying son. As it was, they had to intercede on behalf of their patient because of his mother's display of anger in front of him.

"The good news is that we were able to work with the family and, within a week or so, the situation was much better," she recalls. "But the initial crisis was one of those family meetings that everybody dreads."

Of course, hindsight is always 20/20. What's important is to have your patient and his or her family in your mind's eye early on. If you fear possible landmines, ask a reliable source (whether that is the patient or trusted relative) if they anticipate friction so you're not blindsided. Also, remember that the patient's autonomy remains the most critical issue. You may be supportive of the feelings of family members, but you have to make sure they hear it when Dad says, "I don't want to go on with this cancer treatment." As Hepworth says,

> So often the physician's fear is "What if I get into the room with this family and they start disagreeing about what to do?" There's a lot of anxiety about helping family members control their own anxieties But most families are very polite when they have the opportunity to meet and get information, as long as they feel like they're included.

While physicians can handle the majority of problems, there are those patients who might benefit from collaboration between their physicians and mental health professionals. Dostal, for example, says she has learned that certain issues go beyond her expertise. She welcomes the collaboration with Cohen, in part because patients may have problems that require more attention than her own schedule allows. Also, family issues frequently benefit from a team approach in which members augment each other.

"There are very few doctors who've gone through formal training in family therapy," she says. "And that's an in-depth skill that we frequently identify a need for, but don't necessarily have the tools to carry out appropriately. Having somebody there who can is invaluable."

Collaboration can take many forms, from having a mental health professional on site to developing an affiliation with someone in the community. Some experts propose that each office visit include a therapist for routine screening to determine if underlying issues exist. Obviously, such an approach has its drawbacks. Patients may not accept it, and managed care would certainly look askance at the cost. But the point is that the behavioral component of health issues is so significant that patients may benefit when physicians collaborate with mental health specialists. Therapist Cohen, for example, was able to help a referring physician whose patient suffered from infertility and chronic pain. After a therapy session, she discovered a history of sexual abuse. With this perspective, they were able to discuss the patient's related eating disorder and fear of pregnancy.

No matter what your approach, keep in mind that families often aren't prepared for the stress of a medical crisis. They may appear to be a poorly functioning unit because of the strain and worry. Cohen begins with the assumption that they're doing the best they can and have the best possible intentions. She then sets to work on helping them modify any coping strategies that subvert good patient outcomes.

An essential step is to identify the family's strengths. Even those that are seriously dysfunctional are usually coping in their own fashion. Bloch makes it his business to discover in the first interview with family members just what binds them. It could be: faith and spirituality; humor and an ability to adapt; being good problem-solvers; having connections to an extended family; or rallying as a group even though they don't get along as individuals.

The possibilities are as varied as families themselves. Yet there's usually a point on which you can build communication, whether it's the optimism they share or the feeling of hard luck that plagues them. Even if their belief system is the latter, you can say, "So sorry to hear that. Has it always been bad luck?" They may then acknowledge, "Well, not always." And from that you start to build.

"A question is not simply a question," says Bloch. "It's also a message to the family that you regard them as allies. By saying, 'It's a difficult time, but what strengths help you through tough times?' you're conveying to them: 'Look, you're a resource and I hope to get some help from that.' The most important thing is to think 'family,'" Bloch continues, "and to have the notion that you're not just dealing with an isolated atomic particle. Your patient is connected to others and those connections are important. By thinking about the family and its strengths, you've got tools to bring to a situation. They will be valuable resources."

Bibliography

Christie-Seely J, ed. *Working with the Family in Primary Care: A Systems Approach to Health and Illness.* New York, NY: Praeger Publishers; 1984.

Cohen-Cole S. *The Medical Interview: The Three Function Approach.* St Louis, Mo: Mosby Year Book; 1991.

Council on Medical Education, American Medical Association. CME Report 5-A-98. Enhancing the cultural competence of physicians. In: *Proceedings of the House of Delegates of the American Medical Association: 47th Annual Meeting.* Chicago, Ill: American Medical Association; 1998.

Hahn SR. Families. In: Feldman MD, Christensen JF, eds. *Behavioral Medicine in Primary Care: A Practical Guide.* Stamford, Conn: Appleton & Lange; 1997:57-71.

Helman C. The family culture: a useful concept for family practice. *Fam Med.* 1991;23:376-381.

Kushner K, Meyer D, Hansen M, Bobula J, Hansen J, Pridham K. The family conference: what do patients want? *J Fam Pract.* 1986;23:463-467.

McDaniel S, Campbell TL, Seaburn DB. *Family-Oriented Primary Care.* New York, NY: Springer-Verlag New York; 1990.

Medalie J, Zyzanski S, Langa D, Stange K. The family in family practice: is it a reality? *J Fam Pract.* 1998;46:390-396.

Chapter 5

The Geriatric Patient: Avoid Stereotypes and Increase Understanding

It took a little prodding; but before the visit was over, Dr Ron Amedee's patient—"an 86-year-old jewel of a young lady"—was singing off the same song sheet as her otolaryngologist. Fully conversant and very outgoing, she arrived at his Tulane University School of Medicine office, accompanied by two daughters convinced that their mother wasn't hearing very well. Audio tests showed a natural aging of the inner ear. Amedee considered two different approaches toward conveying this to his patient. He could either launch into a lecture about hearing aids. Or he could make his case by appealing to her as a God-fearing grandmother who loved both her church and her family.

By choosing the latter approach, Amedee was able to gently nudge his patient into acknowledging that she was having a difficult time hearing the minister's sermons each Sunday and also missed much of the conversation at family dinners. In either case, he knew the loss was affecting her quality of life.

"By the time I had made that presentation, she couldn't leave the clinic without having a hearing aid evaluation," he says. "I didn't tell her she needed a hearing aid. *She told me*. If I had forced it on her, she would have put it in the dresser drawer. But by linking the device to two very important things in her life—hearing the Word *and* her family—she couldn't possibly deny herself the opportunity to hear better."

Different yet the Same

Communicating with patients often involves convincing them of what you believe will improve their health. But what happens when that patient is older? What strategies must you then adopt to communicate most effectively?

Talking to elderly patients requires the same basic considerations that should be at play in every patient-physician interaction: Be knowledgeable and forthcoming as well as succinct and clear. Let your words and actions pave the way for questions and opinions. But most important, be respectful. Remember that not every elderly patient is comfortable with today's more informal, "consumer-friendly" practice of medicine. Maybe you've heard the saying, "Don't call me Edna and I won't call you Sonny."

It's worth repeating, given that by the year 2020, one in five Americans will be over the age of 65, compared to one in eight today. What does that mean for you as a physician? You'll be challenged to tailor your basic communication skills, as well as prevent misconceptions about aging from entering your practice. For the lingering stereotypes about seniors don't reflect current scientific research. Indeed, any false assumptions can interfere with your ability to diagnose and treat. Some common mistakes that physicians often make with this patient population include dismissing their symptoms as the result of old age or failing to explain the rationale for their treatment. But perhaps the most egregious error is not to treat at all.

In other words, put aside the mind-set that elderly patients are frustrating and uncooperative or demented and depressed. More often than not, they view their visit with you as a social outing. Don't automatically assume they have a hearing loss and speak too loudly. Don't direct your conversation to their children in the misguided belief the patient must be "confused." Even if signs of frailty are evident, maintaining eye contact and speaking directly to the geriatric patient is as important as paraphrasing what you've said to the caregiver.

Anything less, says Clifford M. Singer, MD, medical director of geriatric psychiatry at Oregon Health Sciences University, "is generally insulting and sometimes makes going to a doctor an unpleasant or humiliating experience. But if an older person is directly engaged and understands the reason for the visit, then it's often pleasurable. When you have better rapport, you just get better information and do a better job teaching."

Older adults are as diverse in their problems and perceptions as are any other group. Yes, there are difficulties with deafness, dementia, and, certainly, disease. However, as Singer writes in *Behavioral Medicine in Primary Care: A Practical Guide*, a person's temperament (energy and intensity) remains remarkably stable throughout adult life, while his or her personality (learned behavior patterns) undergoes refinement.

Although mental illnesses and neurodegenerative diseases take their toll, most elderly persons remain actively curious, even though there may be predictable changes in intellect. For example, they may process information and learn new tasks more slowly or not cope as well with distraction. However, some would say that the elderly are *more* cooperative as patients, even reluctant to report their health problems because they view them as an inevitable part of aging. Also, because they vary widely in cultural backgrounds, educational or economic levels, and health status, they (as do all patients) bring many views and experiences to the medical encounter.

But threaded throughout that plurality are commonalities. Like most of us, older people want to be viewed as individuals with their own unique responses to disease. Also, like many of us, they feel, look, and even see themselves as younger than their calendar years. As humorist Mark Russell once opined, "Inside every older person is a younger person saying, 'What the hell happened?'"

A Heightened Awareness

Being aware of any communication barriers between you and your elderly patients is the first helpful step you can take toward resolving them. Authors Scott Mader, MD, and Amasa Ford, MD—writing in *The Medical Interview: Clinical Care, Education, and Research*—identify common hurdles that fall into three areas: physical (hearing impairment, dementia, delirium, and depression.); psychosocial (ageism, education, language, culture, and transference or countertransference); and "other" (financial and time limitations, knowledge deficits, and fear of a loss of independence).

In general, you won't need special expertise to deal with those patients in their early 60s and 70s, who often are still robust and healthy, fully independent, and functioning. If they have hearing, visual, or cognitive impairment, it's generally mild, unless caused by a degenerative disease. But those in their 80s and 90s may require your closest attention as a group because of their frailties. Your interactions with them may take additional time and patience, with you slowing the pace to make sure you've been heard and, more important, understood. Mader goes on to suggest that what you ask *yourself* with every encounter affects the outcome as much as what you ask the patient. For example:

"Can they hear you?"

"Do they understand what you're saying (barring any language barriers or dementia)?"

"Do they feel comfortable sharing their problems?"

"Is there enough time? Do you appear unhurried and interested?"

"Do you recognize transference and countertransference issues that may impair communication (such as a patient reluctant to discuss sexual concerns with a doctor who reminds him of his granddaughter?)"

"Are you sensitive to the patient's chief complaint and to issues regarding diagnostic tests and independence?"

According to Bob G. Knight, PhD, MD, Merle H. Ensinger associate professor of gerontology and psychology at the University of Southern California's Andrus Gerontology Center, the first mistake many physicians make when it comes to their interactions with older patients is that they overlook their divergent life histories and outlooks. He suggests framing the encounter in light of that patient's life experience. For example, what was the world like when he or she became an adult?

What values governed their generation? "Being able to show knowledge of things that happened before you were born demonstrates that you can kind of identify with their frame of reference," Knight says.

Paving the Way

Effective communication with your elderly patients also depends partly on your staff as well as your practice environment. To smooth the way, especially with the first visit, have seniors fill out any questionnaires prior to the visit. This allows them—and their caregivers—to provide complete data. If forms are completed in the office, structure them for quick and easy responses. Or have your nurse or other health care professional assist the patient with each form. That gives you more time to explore the patients' concerns, time that would otherwise be spent collecting their medical history.

Always encourage older patients to address problems that are specific to your specialty, although you'll want to hear about any heart or chronic health conditions. But if you're the otolaryngologist treating hearing loss, or the gasteroenterologist probing for colon cancer, let the patient know you need to focus on the problem that concerns your specialty.

Further, urge your patients to show you what pills or supplements they take. One of the biggest problems physicians face in treating older patients is their multiple medications and the variety of specialists who prescribe them. Edith McFadden, MD, an allergist at the University of Chicago's Pritzger School of Medicine, makes it a point to always query about over-the-counter medications her patients have purchased, as well as any prescriptive drugs they might be sampling from others. Among her elderly clients, she finds that sharing pills is a recurring issue, particularly for persons living in the close quarters of a retirement community.

"Even if they tell me, 'No I don't do that sort of thing,' at least I've touched on the topic," McFadden says. "Then I can say, 'That's good because it's a dangerous thing to do.' Even if they feel embarrassed or don't tell me [the truth], at least I have a chance to reinforce that they shouldn't be doing it."

A Conducive Atmosphere

Because environmental conditions can impair communication and rapport, factors that might detract from the encounter deserve special attention. Remember that older people are more sensitive to glare and are less able to discriminate among shades and colors. For example, if you sit in front of a window with the sun behind you, it may be difficult for your patient to see your features, make eye contact, or, if necessary, read your lips. Conversely, if you place yourself at eye level, your patients are more likely to register your words. And they may even think you're spending more time with them than the clock suggests.

Also, noise can be especially disruptive to elderly adults, many of whom have poor hearing or impaired cognition. Up to 40% of persons 65 or older experience hearing loss, according to the American Academy of Otolaryngology, Head and Neck Surgery. Other statistics suggest that, by age 79, 50% of people have significant impairment. Because older adults often can't hear voices when there's a lot of background noise, make sure that you're not only in a face-to-face encounter but also in a quiet room.

Don't resort to shouting. It only distorts sound and may make you appear angry. Since presbycusis diminishes hearing in the higher range, speak in low tones. Also, don't drop your voice at the end of sentences, but pause between them. If your patient doesn't understand, repeat the statement using different words rather than overarticulating.

Your office and nursing staff are excellent eyes and ears for you concerning the health status of all patients, especially those who are older. They're often the sounding boards for problems these patients may not want to "bother" the doctor with. While staff members can't delegate your duties, they can allay concerns and observe what goes on in the waiting and exam rooms. They see how much trouble patients have getting dressed, following directions, or walking down the hall. Was he so confused this morning that he tried to leave before seeing the physician? Did her gait look right? Did either of them have difficulty making a next appointment?

Most important, your staff steps in where you leave off, as long as you've paved the way by giving them credibility. For example, if your patient needs to take better control of his or her diabetes, you might suggest a talk with your nurse, leading with:

> *"We have somebody here who knows a whole lot more about how to manage diabetes at home than I do. It might be good for you to talk with her (or him) before you leave today. Then, when questions arise, she (or he) is often easier to reach than I am."*

On the Alert

History-taking will no doubt focus on your patient's health. But you should also be alert to any information about personal relationships, responses to stress, or attitudes toward the family. It's essential, say experts, that you determine the health beliefs and other expectations of every patient because they vary according to ethnic and cultural backgrounds or experience and age.

Also, even though someone may be past the age at which familial conditions typically appear, a family history can still indicate the likelihood that either the patient or his or her caretaker could develop a specific disease. Similarly, you'll want to know if your patient is the caregiver for someone else. In any case, such discussions are a good springboard for conversations about an individual's experiences with and attitudes toward disease and death. You may learn, for example, that he doesn't want to be placed in a nursing home or that she wants an advance directive.

Myriad diagnostic tools and methodology—either inside or outside the office—can help you progressively measure an older patient's cognitive and other functions. However, you can get a very preliminary assessment even as you enter the exam room. Is this someone who is going to be difficult to engage? Do you have to use nonverbal cues to engage his or her attention? Is he or she anxious enough to need their hand held? You'll determine quickly if your patient is spry, lively, hears and speaks well, or processes information easily. If so, you won't have to make many adjustments in your approach to communication.

An Altered Approach

Flexibility should be the byword of each encounter with elderly patients, with you willing to deviate from the usual interview structure to learn more in less time. Resist your initial impulses to lead with questions about ongoing problems from previous visits. That approach often leaves individuals until the end of the appointment to articulate their current concerns, which may vary greatly from your agenda, suggests Barbara Gastel, MD, author of the National Institute on Aging's (NIA) *Working With Your Older Patient: A Clinician's Handbook*. Instead, open each encounter with:

> *"How can I help you most at this visit?"* or

> *"What's been happening since we last talked?"*

From there, it's a matter of pacing the interview, keeping in mind that older patients may need extra time to formulate their answers and organize their thoughts. You'll want to take a deep breath and move at the pace the patient establishes.

By consciously slowing your speech and giving the individual time to respond, Knight suggests, you'll get through the interview more efficiently than if you're talking too fast and then have to repeat your message or answer a number of questions to clarify things. By slowing the motion, you're showing the patient that you're willing to give him or her as much time as necessary.

Research shows that physicians tend to interrupt within seconds to turn to other matters. So give your patients wide berth. If they have difficulty with open-ended questions, revert to inquiries that need either a yes or no response or a simple choice answer. Remember also that many older patients resent a structured encounter that uses formatted questions, instead of focusing on what the patient wants to discuss.

"If you don't address their chief complaint, which may not be the most significant medically, they won't comply with anything else you recommend," says Lisa Gwyther, MSW, director of the family support program at Duke University's Aging Center. "Even though you think someone's heart condition is more serious than their foot pain, you've got to address the foot pain first."

Indeed, physicians are often so involved with reviewing various organ systems that they miss the questions critical to many older patients: sleep loss, incontinence, falls, depression, dizziness, loss of energy, and fatigue are passed over when physicians are rushed or patients are embarrassed.

In addition, unlike younger individuals who have well-defined symptoms, elderly adults often have nonspecific complaints they can't describe. Or they experience atypical presentations—the heart attack that doesn't occur with left-sided pain, but instead causes confusion or lesser pain. Since older adults suffer multiple chronic ailments, the most important questions you may pose are those that ferret out the acuity of a problem.

"How fast has this changed?" or

"Has this happened before?"

If you don't see your elderly patients as individuals and focus only on the chronic nature of illness in older adults, you run the risk of being less vigilant about their acute problems. For their part, older adults are often daunted by the complex, interrelated medical conditions that now mark their lives, as well as the confusing labyrinth of specialists and instructions they have to endure. And they may have difficulty sorting it out for you.

"Many older people don't understand, or they get frustrated, because they're used to the fact that when they were younger they'd go to the doctor, get treated and they'd get well," says Gwyther. "And the one thing we know about getting older is it may take longer."

Toward Optimal Understanding

Unless there's a doctor in the house, your older patients probably are unfamiliar with your medical lexicon, so leave the jargon for your staff and concentrate on words and phrases familiar to a lay audience. Hypertension is "high blood pressure," carcinoma is "cancer," and a myocardial infarction remains a "heart attack."

Since they may not be acquainted with such concepts such as "helplines" and "support groups," or know how to "network," be prepared to translate these expressions. Also, use visual metaphors and analogies generously, especially if they apply to something from the past. Further, it's never a good idea to overload older patients with blocks of information, but better to break messages into small pieces.

When you want to take the interview in a new direction, alert the patient by pausing briefly or raising your voice slightly. Mader and his colleague suggest simply saying: "Now I'd like to ask you questions about your heart." Throughout the conversation, remember to monitor the patient's comprehension of what you've said, asking him or her to repeat it in their own words. Also, if they seem to have misconceptions or inadequate information that may make it difficult for them to follow your treatment regimen, you may have to gently correct their thinking:

"We used to believe that, but our research now shows it isn't so." or

"We're learning that there's more that can be done."

In the same vein, make sure you tell elderly patients what to expect and when they might feel better or know that the treatment is working. That's often a missed topic. Also make use of factsheets, pamphlets, and audiotapes or videos to extend your communication beyond the office.

Particularly when the discussion is about surgery, follow-up materials often are available from your professional society. These can orient a person as to what to expect, even if you've already laid the groundwork. (You might even suggest the NIA's *Talking With Your Doctor: A Guide for Older People* as a tool to help your patients talk to you.)

The caveat, of course, is that written materials won't suffice if an individual isn't literate or fluent in the language. If that's the case, you may have to use diagrams or drawings to clarify concepts or give the materials to relatives who do read. In fact, having a third person with whom to talk things over, or who can take notes about treatment and medications, is often a good idea. Just suggest to the patient that two heads are better than one. You think it would be helpful if someone else participated in the conversation.

This is even more necessary when your patient is very old, unless the individual is in exceptional health, functioning and independent. However, most people in their 80s and 90s, Gwyther suggests, have some functional or cognitive impairment that may impede their own understanding of their problems, not to mention your progress with them. When dealing alone with someone in a frail condition, it may be harder to make the right diagnosis or to see your treatment plan executed.

Having an interview with family or a caregiver, Singer suggests, can help you complete the picture. Begin by establishing the patient's condition with everyone involved. Then spend time with the patient to assess his or her neurologic and mental status and to hear any concerns they may be afraid to mention in front of others. Meanwhile, a staff member can interview the caregiver for a detailed history and description of any symptoms they may not want to share in the patient's presence.

Singer tells the story of meeting with a patient in the early stages of Alzheimer's disease, along with his wife. The physician picked up signals that the man wanted to talk to him alone. So against the protests of a protective and worried spouse, he sequestered himself with his patient. Outside her presence, the man, still bright, poured forth with an elaborate delusional scheme as to how he lost his wealth and how ashamed he was about it. Such was not the case (as his wife and attorney had already attested). But by spending those intimate moments with the patient, Singer was able to glean very dramatic information about where this man was headed, including having intense suicidal thoughts.

In any case, you want to give each of your older patients ample time to share their stories and include them in any decision making about their care. Also, since patients sometimes aren't comfortable expressing certain concerns—the death of a close relative or friend, for example—give them an opening before you finish your evaluation:

"Is there anything else you'd like to discuss?"

Respect Your Elders

When you can communicate effectively with your elderly patients, their anxieties are lessened, which in turn enables their questions and concerns to be addressed. For your part, you may enjoy your interactions with this generation a bit more because it becomes a more human connection. And why not? These are the people who paved the way for us.

It might not be a bad idea to take the lead from Thomas Perls, MD, director of the New England Centenarian Study, and author of *Living to 100: Lessons in Living to*

Your Maximum Potential at Any Age, which chronicles life lessons of those who've crossed the century mark as vibrant, independent, functional, and healthy individuals.

"When you come across an older, but completely cognitively intact and healthy individual, you need to relate as you would to any other adult patient," Perls says. "None of this infantilization or assumptions about what they can't do because they, in my estimation, would continue to have a very keen interest in their health and preserving their cognitive and physical function.

"You can't assume that what you might prescribe in terms of activities, medications, or a care plan would be any different for these people than it would be for a younger person."

Bibliography

Anderson E. Getting through to elderly patients. *Geriatrics 46*. 1991;No. 5:74-76.

Anderson E. How not to talk to elderly patients. *Geriatrics 45*. 1990;No. 1:84-85.

Gastel B. *Working with Your Older Patient: A Clinician's Handbook*. Bethesda, Md: National Institute on Aging, National Institutes of Health; 1994.

Mader S, Ford A. The geriatric interview. In: Lipkin M Jr, Putnam SM, Lazare A, eds. *The Medical Interview: Clinical Care, Education and Research*. New York, NY: Springer-Verlag New York; 1995:221-235.

Mungas D. In-office mental status testing: a practical guide. *Geriatrics 46*. 1991;No. 7:54-63.

Perls T, Hutter Silver M, Lauerman JF. *Living to 100: Lessons in Living to Your Maximum Potential at Any Age*. New York, NY: Basic Books; 1999.

Singer C, Jones S, Ganzini L. Older patients. In: Feldman MD, Christensen, JF, eds. *Behavioral Medicine in Primary Care: A Practical Guide*. Stamford, Conn: Appleton & Lange; 1997:89-96.

Slocum H. Not him again! Thoughts on coping with irritating elderly patients. *Geriatrics 44*. 1989;No. 10:75-84.

Smith R, Engel G. *The Patient's Story*. Boston, Mass: Little, Brown and Company; 1996.

Talking With Your Doctor: A Guide for Older Patients. Bethesda, Md: National Institute on Aging, National Institutes of Health; 1994.

Chapter 6

The Difficult Patient: Overcome Obstacles to Care

Wouldn't it be great to take creative license with your medical practice? Think of the patients—your own cast of characters—who'd act like you want them to act, move like you want them to move, and emote like you want them to emote.

Wouldn't it be wonderful if everyone took perfect direction, no matter what role he or she was cast to play? Think how smoothly the drama would unfold if the actors followed each syllable of your advice.

Unfortunately, physicians don't have creative license; and most patients can't be moved like actors on stage, even though many of them, mercifully, will heed direction. In the real world of medicine, people aren't always compliant, cooperative, grateful, or polite.

In fact, among the people in your caseload, you probably can find your share of "difficult" patients—those who kindle in you the same ire that actors inspire in directors by being frustrating to direct. But who's to blame here?

Experts tell us that the tense scenes between physicians and patients are rarely the fault of one person but often are created by miscommunication, bad communication, or no communication between individuals. That is, you have a bigger role in each patient's drama than you've imagined since everyone carries baggage into an encounter. Yes, even you.

Maybe your father was an alcoholic and now you have a visceral reaction to patients who abuse liquor. Or your mother never controlled her diabetes so you won't tolerate patients who can't either.

Physical conditions. Attitudes and personality traits. Your own history. Any number of issues can create communication barriers between physicians and patients. Any number of situations can trigger your darkest thoughts and reactions while they do nothing to your colleagues.

"It's not possible to practice medicine without being personal because it's a human interaction," says Wendy Levinson, MD, chief of general internal medicine, Pritzger School of Medicine, University of Chicago. "We're not robots. We bring our humanness to every encounter, with every single patient. It's powerful, effective and very important. It's the basis of trust, respect and belief our patients have in us."

Eyes of a Beholder

Knowing who you are as a person and integrating that wisdom into your performance as a professional may be the most important challenge you face in medicine. For interfacing effectively with patients is the very task, on any given day, with any given visit, that gives clinical work its satisfaction and meaning. Otherwise, say experts, practicing medicine can become a mere technical endeavor that eventually turns boring and even leads to burnout. As one physician notes, "You kind of lose a personal interest and investment in the work of doctoring."

Managed care certainly hasn't made the task easier. Instead, it has shuffled the cards in terms of decision making, putting limits on your time and choices. Granted, many would suggest that a system designed to make health care more cost effective isn't all bad because it forces physicians to be more efficient. But physicians complain that the deck is often stacked against them when they want to spend sufficient time with patients who seem difficult to talk to or even treat. With office visits now averaging 20 minutes or less, there's little wiggle room to address big issues or the concerns of individuals who may distrust medicine—and you.

But the reassuring news is that when it comes to understanding your reactions to your patients and dealing with their reactions to you, you don't have to just play the cards you're dealt. You can strengthen your hand by developing a series of skills that help you recognize your emotional hot buttons—and the people pushing them.

Unfortunately, difficult patients don't present with one set of symptoms or personality traits. In fact, the common thread is not who they are so much as what distress they can cause in others. For starters, there's anxiousness, anger, and an all-around sense of being overwhelmed and frustrated by the behavior. You may recognize the general queasiness in the pit of your stomach when you see the name on the appointment list. These are often the patients whose folders are fat because they utilize so many services.

Depending on the ire they elicit, difficult patients are called every name from "heartsink" to "hateful," the latter described by James E. Groves, MD, in the April 26, 1978, *New England Journal of Medicine*. They're the ones with whom physicians have more than an occasional personality clash.

Dependent clingers have no discernible medical illness but are overtly needy and evoke aversion in their physicians. *Entitled demanders* use intimidation and guilt to control, while eliciting rage and fear in practitioners. *Manipulative help rejecters* exhibit a pessimism that increases in direct proportion to a physician's effectiveness.

They stimulate guilt and inadequacy in their providers. *Self-destructive deniers* relish their own dissolution, delighting in defeating any help. They arouse malice and even the secret wish that this person would "die and get it over with."

While Groves' stereotypes may be an apt depiction, others suggest that identifying another person as the problem only places blame. Instead, it's more fruitful to reframe the difficulties with specific patients as a product of the interaction rather than the individual. It's more productive to look at both dance partners—since it takes two to tango.

Certainly, there are those persons who would drive most doctors to distraction. They're often the somatizers who show up with symptoms that lack any demonstrable organic cause or exceed the expectations of objective medical findings. Or they're the borderline personalities who view the world in terms of good guys and bad guys. On any given day you could be the nurturing angel—or the persecuting devil.

But, for the most part, the people who give physicians trouble are found somewhere in the physicians' own past. Perhaps you can identify with the sketch of the physician, the patient, and their respective family trees crowding the examining room. Sound familiar? If so, it's not surprising since many encounters become problematic the moment your past experiences come in contact with your patient's present circumstances.

Perhaps you don't hesitate to work with drug addicts, but passive-aggressive patients are your nemesis. Your mother was so much more controlling than your father that the interaction between them was always difficult to watch, so now you find it equally hard to meet people whose situation parallels theirs. Or your father died of a heart attack and you have a difficult time working up men with cardiac symptoms. You go through a lot of second-guessing each time.

Alcoholics. Obese people. Dependent, demanding, or drug-addicted patients. Difficulty is definitely in the eyes of the beholder. To paraphrase the old bromide, what's one physician's trauma may not be another's trouble. Instead, every practitioner has multiple demands and personal agendas that can get between him or her and a patient. The trick is to leave them outside the examination room or, better yet, deal with them so they become a powerful resource in your dealings with others.

"We are all wounded healers in one aspect or another. And our wounds are not only the sources of our pain but at times, they're the source of our compassion and strength," says Richard R. Irons, MD, staff physician, Professionals in Crisis Program, Menninger Clinic. "Our goal as doctors should be to cleanse ourselves of as many of those thoughts as possible so we can truly be present in the moment."

Making Peace with the Past

There's a potent message to be found in the Biblical reference, "Physician, heal thyself." For the secret in taking care of patients, particularly those who cause you consternation and grief, is in recognizing that your responsibility stops at the medical water's edge. That is, you can care for their health needs, but you can't care for their behavior. You can, however, change your own behavior.

In fact, how well physicians connect with patients depends largely on the awareness they have of their own past experiences and their ability to corral them into a resource. Writing in the August 13, 1997, *Journal of the American Medical Association*, Dennis Novack, MD, and his colleagues suggest that this is where the science of medicine merges with the art. Physicians learn many skills to elicit facts, arrive at diagnoses, and influence decision making. But being effective in using them depends entirely on their skills in recognizing and dealing with their own issues.

That is, feelings and attitudes that aren't acknowledged can interfere with one's ability to communicate empathetically. They can be a hindrance in conversations, precluding or distorting discussions about sensitive topics such as death. And they can change the dynamic of your participation to over- or underinvolvement.

Conversely, by appreciating where you've been and how you've gotten there, you can be more effective in your encounters. Novack refers to it as physicians "calibrating" themselves—that is, becoming more effectual in their efforts to be the instruments of diagnosis and therapy they've been called by other researchers.

Indeed, as with everyone, the tapestry of a physician's emotional life is woven with many different threads. For instance, core beliefs and attitudes, which make up your personal philosophy, can profoundly determine how you listen to a patient's story and lend empathy and advice.

Similarly, sociocultural influences include the many factors—education, income, and social class—that shape you. As disparate as they may be from your patient's, they form the basis of your attitudes toward acceptable illness behavior and other emotionally charged issues. They also influence how you delineate information and interact with others.

Further, your gender is a core element of your identity, which also affects your professional development, clinical decision making, and relationship with your patients. Novack suggests, for example, that studies have shown women physicians engage in more preventive services and screen patients at a higher rate than men. They also conduct longer visits and use more patient-centered communication strategies than male physicians, who are more likely to provide answers that are less technical than the questions actually posed by their female patients. In any case, physician attitudes and expectations, as well as their interactive styles, are affected by the disparate ways men and women develop psychologically.

Similarly, a physician's behaviors and attitudes about intimacy and conflict resolution, among other issues, are rooted in his or her family of origin. Patterns pass through generations, with people learning first from family about communicating illness and responding to distress.

The classic example is the physician who has a hard time with anger, fearing it as potentially destructive. Or maybe this individual is conflict avoidant because he or she had a bad experience being yelled at earlier in life. Even though the mind says, "I did nothing wrong," emotionally this person thinks he or she did.

Another physician, facing the same tirade, may not see it as destructive, having grown up in a family where the expression was commonplace but not destructive. In that case, the physician might even enjoy stepping up to the challenge of dealing with someone's rage.

In any case, ignoring emotional patterns of any sort can hinder your relationships with patients by distorting your perceptions of them and their families. When you don't recognize the connection between the behaviors you see in an individual and those that may be in your past, you open yourself to feelings of inadequacy, loss of control, and even fear of hurting the person.

Instead, working through the meshugas in your life should help you understand your own personal biases, relieve any emotional baggage, and assist you in gaining a new perspective on your "difficult" patients.

How do you get from here to there? Through a lot of soul-searching and support. More specifically, there are any number of paths to take in finding your strengths and building on them. There are any number of questions to ask in exploring how your attitudes were shaped and why you respond the way you do to certain situations. For example, if you're afraid of the anger in your patient—or even that it will show up in you—Novack suggests probing with these kinds of questions:

> *"What sorts of patients elicit an angry reaction in me?"*
>
> *"What work situation usually makes me angry and why?"*
>
> *"What are my usual responses to my own anger and the anger of others? (eg, Do I overreact, placate, blame others, suppress my own feelings, become superreasonable?)"*
>
> *"What are the underlying feelings when I become angry (eg, feeling rejected, humiliated, unworthy)?"*
>
> *"Where did I learn my responses to anger?"*

You can ponder every aspect of your attitudes with simple questions that focus on your development. Queries that help you identify the culture influencing your past or the values you liked or disliked from your heritage focus attention on the sociocultural influences in your life. Similarly, you gain insight when you ask what messages you received early in life about sex or gender roles and how those attitudes affect the way you communicate with male versus female patients. Further, there's a gold mine of information about your family's influence that you can pan for with questions, such as the following, suggested by Novack:

"What role did I have in my family?"

"How might I be relating these roles in my work environment?"

"What lessons did I learn from my family about the nature of relationships, about the nature of caregiving, and about acceptable responses to illness?"

"What kinds of patients might I be likely to associate with family members?"

In any case, from reflection to psychotherapy, the goal is to choose an option—perhaps keeping a journal or videotaping your interactions for critique—that fits your personal style.

But the best approaches may be the ones you pursue with your colleagues. As Ronald M. Epstein, MD, and his coauthors suggest in the October 1993 issue of *The Journal of Family Practice*, group dynamics expose individual physicianrs to the issues of their colleagues while providing a forum for support and common ground.

You're probably already familiar with family-of-origin groups, which utilize the concepts of intergenerational family therapy to focus on a physician's past and present family issues in terms of the patient relationship. During group sessions, each physician utilizes a genogram or family tree as a graphic means to access some of the stories, traditions, attributes, and myths that are part of his or her own background. From there the discussion centers on the strengths, rather than shortcomings, in that individual's family-of-origin so he or she can explore difficulties or blind spots.

Similarly, Balint groups, a format developed by Michael and Enid Balint in the 1950s, gives practicing physicians an intense small-group forum in which to present difficult cases while exploring any feelings that could interfere with those encounters. Often incorporating family therapy concepts, the sessions are generally led by a psychiatrist, psychologist, or social worker.

But those are only two formats among many—including personal awareness groups that focus on difficult cases and other workplace issues in the context of relationships—providing for self-discovery. Professional organizations such as the

American Academy on Physician and Patient (AAPP) offer discussions on personal awareness in its interpersonal skills courses.

Workshops concerning difficult clinician-patient relationships are also among the many sessions that the Bayer Institute for Health Care Communication has initiated since its inception in 1987. A nonprofit organization, the institute's mission is to enhance quality of care by improving clinician-patient communication. It does so through various approaches, including research and advocacy, as well as training of physicians to teach others.

Among the workshops the institute sponsors, the session on difficult clinician-patient relationships examines various patterns of interaction that can cause some of the greatest communication challenges for physicians. The course can be taken for continuing medical education (CME), meeting the criteria for Category I of the Physician's Recognition Award of the American Medical Association.

Whichever structure one chooses, the same caveat applies: Self-awareness is a process that lasts a lifetime and isn't an end in itself. Susan McDaniel, coauthor of the book *Family-Oriented Primary Care*, belongs to a group in which some members first crafted their own genograms in 1982. Today they put up the schematics, along with the family trees of patients, to discuss individual cases as well as personal issues associated with being a physician.

As a psychologist, McDaniel can't think of a time when she won't be tethered to such a support network. Like her physician-colleagues, she brings what she learns during those weekly sessions into her other interactions.

"Once physicians have done this," she says, "I think it's hard for them not to think, when they have a case they're having difficulty with, 'Does this have anything to do with my background?' or 'Is it overloaded with some of my own family issues?'

"In a group they can brainstorm. They can say, 'Maybe reacting to your patient as if he were your father isn't the best way to go. What other ways are there to be helpful to this person?' They really need someplace to talk no matter how experienced or talented they are."

Taking Your Cues

Physicians are unique in the internal cues they develop to alert them to the dynamics, good or bad, of every interview. But there are generic warning signs, McDaniel suggests in her book, to tell you when the conversation is going south and you need to change the direction.

Often physicians find themselves prescribing the same treatments or taking the same educational steps repeatedly when there's no improvement. The boredom, sadness, or anger is out of proportion to the problem. Their hearts sink when they see certain names on the scheduling sheets. Worse yet, they limit the time spent with those patients, finding excuses to shorten visits or punt phone requests to others.

Other experts would say to watch for changes in your gut feeling or a shift in the atmosphere when this person walks in the door. Unlike normal conversations with your patients, during these interactions, the two of you are constantly interrupting each other or covering the same ground repeatedly. Particularly when the individual has a personality disorder, you feel bad or devalued after the visit.

In any case, whether you're restless or resentful, your reactions are telling you that something's going on here that doesn't happen with other patients. Is this person's seeming reactions really directed at you or at the disease? Did you truly mess up or is the system interfering with both of you? It's time to pause, ponder the emotional data you're collecting, and use them to diagnose why. As Geoffrey Gordon, MD, associate director for clinical education and research, Bayer Health Institute for Healthcare Communication, suggests:

> It's those times when you need to step back and say, "You know I'm off my pace with this patient. Something's happening here and I need to think in the terms of where could the problem lie and what should I do next?" The trick is to recognize early that difficulties are on the horizon rather than waiting until the canoe is over the falls.

Small Steps for Big Outcomes

Your emotions in difficult encounters are matched only by those of your patients. They may have psychosocial stresses or even psychiatric diagnoses that determine the nature of their symptoms and response to treatment. You've probably seen an array of defenses that make these people less pleasant and more pugnacious, seductive, angry, and/or hostile.

Often these patients have expectations based on memories of every patient-physician interaction they've ever witnessed. Someone's mother, for instance, suffered cancer at the hands of a physician who seemed cold and dispassionate. Fill in the blank and you have history and its accompanying projections walking into the examining room with someone's medical status and inability to tell his or her story. As Irons suggests:

The difficult patient comes in with pain and its attendant cousins, which are anger, frustration, tiredness, boredom, impatience and doubt. All of those cousins are in the room with you and you've got to sort through them. Remember, the reason you're there is to hear both the biological and non-biological aspects of this person's pain. That's where the difficulty begins.

While your ultimate goal is to provide care, you may have to help this person lay down as many defenses as possible to get to that point. For dealing with the difficult patient-clinician interaction starts with identifying the other emotions in the room—the ones driving this individual. As one physician suggests, the emotions that both you and your patient exhibit are like weather systems. There's nothing inherently right or wrong in them. But if you're on the receiving end of a rough front—your patient is deeply sad or angry—you may want to use the situation like a weather report. By allowing this person to vent his or her emotions, you decrease the intensity of the storm, making room for a new front to move in.

You'll get further faster by understanding the cause of someone's behavior rather than prematurely lumping that individual into one category or another. For instance, what are the reasons, suggests Howard Beckman, MD, that one patient seems angry or another is silent? What's causing this individual to be demanding while that one counters every suggestion with "yes . . . but." Writing in *Behavioral Medicine in Primary Care: A Practical Guide*, Beckman suggests those four portraits as the most common harbingers of other, more deep-seeded problems in patients.

You may be broadsided by an angry patient's stony silence, piercing stares, or utter refusal to shake hands. Or you experience the withdrawal and nervous habits, lost eye contact, and verbal interaction from someone who is silent.

Perhaps you've encountered the poor attention, frustration, or anxiety exhibited by a demanding individual. Or you've had a number of "yes . . . but" patients whose demeanors became marked by a shift in posture when the conversation turned to evaluation and treatment. When the dialogue is serious, they become quiet, offering no solutions and volunteering little outside of "I'd like to do that, but. . . ."

While those "symptoms" could send you into a personal frenzy over what you've said or done, the diagnoses are more involved and often have nothing to do with you. Even though you take your patient's anger as a personal swipe at your performance, eliciting all sorts of doubts and defenses, it may not be directed at you at all. Instead, your failures and foibles might be one reason on a list of many—from problems with medications to those of referral physicians—for that anger.

Or someone's silence frustrates you because it's a reminder of your uncle's reticence about his own chest pains that ultimately led to his death. In this case, however, the silence between you could indicate a number of diagnoses, including depression, passive personality, fear of authority, or denial of a disease.

Similarly, when it comes to "yes . . . but" patients, you may start by eagerly offering suggestions which, to your dismay, are either rejected or agreed to and never carried out. Any number of forces may be at work, including the fact that your treatment plan hasn't taken into account this person's perspective or that he or she has a highly controlling family. Disagreeing or dealing with you simply doesn't cross your patient's mind.

Further, while you feel rejected, humiliated, or blamed when your patient starts making demands, your defensiveness may be missing the mark. Yes, this person could be dissatisfied with your treatment plan. But Beckman suggests that other reasons—from concern over the diagnosis to fear that managed care is forcing your decision—could be driving his or her demands.

Yet you won't know unless you ask, for instance, that the person who wants an MRI to exclude an aneurysm is adamant because an emergency room physician once told his or her brother not to worry about his headache and later he died from an aneurysm.

Or you're miffed when you're patient demands the same high-tech test because you know that the HMO frowns on it for such early stage back pain. Unless you ask, you won't know that this person is frightened about being paralyzed. Instead, by soliciting input, you may be able to negotiate another solution:

> *"I can see that this seems to be really important to you to have an MRI. I want to reassure you that if one is indicated, I will order it. But it would really help me to understand what you think it would show us right now."*

In so doing, you're acknowledging the person's emotions while soliciting his or her perspective. Questions such as "How had you hoped I could help you?" provide someone with an opportunity to vent any frustrations over your decision making. The answer may even lighten your load should you learn, as Beckman suggests, that this person's complaint may have been about a sore hip but his or her request is for a cane—not replacement surgery.

Difficult situations are exacerbated when patients view physicians as sitting on the opposite side of the table—or, worse, on the same side of the disease. As Barry Egener, MD, medical director of the Northwest Center for Physician-Patient Communication and president of the AAPP, observes:

> You can't get to the medical issues until you deal with emotions directly. This is scary for doctors because they worry that they're opening Pandora's box. If they talk about emotions, they're afraid the interview will get out of control. But the reality is that talking about emotions can diffuse them.

Whether you think of it as developing a partnership or building an alliance, the idea is to dispel any conflict that might be undermining the therapeutic relationship. It doesn't matter if you're dealing with raw emotions or dissipating disagreements, as in every encounter your ultimate goal is to build trust.

That could be a tall order since practitioners spend a great deal of time projecting onto patients what they think they're feeling instead of asking them. What's more disheartening for patients, according to research by Anthony L. Suchman, MD, and his colleagues, published in the February 26, 1997, issue of the *Journal of the American Medical Association*, is that physicians repeatedly miss or terminate opportunities to be empathetic.

Even when patients, who seldom verbalize their emotions directly, offer lead-ins, clinicians allow those signals to pass, returning instead to the topic at hand. The authors surmise that there are many factors at play, including the physician's own lack of sensitivity and fear of tapping into someone's suffering. But the real problem, they add, is that medical training imbues in clinicians certain attitudes and behaviors that make cultivating objective data more important than cultivating relationships.

How does that affect your interactions with difficult individuals? Failing to listen for their real concerns keeps you fixated on problems that don't exist, while problems that do exist remain unfixed.

Yet, if you're like your colleagues, you've probably stuttered your way to another topic or used vacuities to deal with the one at hand. Instead, you need to find a common lens through which both of you can look or, if that's not possible, get enough exposure to your patient's point of view so you have a clear picture of the situation.

More specifically, no matter what emotions are in the air, you want to: point out the problem, elicit your patient's perspective, empathize with this person's experience, explain what needs to be done, and respond to his or her cues. Egener suggests five emotion-handling skills to deal directly with overtones that suggest difficulties:

- *Reflection.* Name the emotion to your patient so he or she sees that you're interested:

  "You seem upset."

- *Validation.* Explain that you understand why he or she may be upset and show that you're vested in the situation:

  "I can understand that you'd be angry if I left you sitting in this room half-undressed for half an hour." or

  "I can understand that anyone who feels that he or she needs that particular drug and doesn't get it might be upset."

- **Support.** Ease the immediate stress with both verbal and nonverbal responses— patting the shoulder or handing out tissue:

  "I'd like to help."

- **Partnership.** Offer specific help to move this person forward, especially if the first part of the encounter was rough:

  "I wonder what we could do to get over this awkward beginning to our interview."

- **Respect.** Honor the emotional resources of your patient as well as his or her autonomy:

  "You've done a really good job dealing with this chronic illness." or

  "I want you to know that regardless of your choice, I'm going to be there to help you with it."

In any case, you want to pace the interview rather than jumping in impulsively and risk mimicking your patient's behavior. Instead, by slowing your own delivery— delaying responses and letting go of the muscle tension in your face, jaw, and gut— you can begin to clear the air.

Also, when this same person challenges your decisions, the other thing you want to lose is your defensiveness. It only escalates everyone's mood. Instead of ignoring the information your patient shares about the new lower dose of the medication she's taking for her libido, it's more fruitful to acknowledge:

"Well, I'm glad that you shared that with me. I didn't know. Let's look at it together."

Such an approach disarms the patient while giving you an opening to make your case—in this instance, to convince her that sticking with the current prescription is the best regimen. Similarly, drawing boundaries for yourself, whether they cover the way you practice medicine or relate to your patients outside the office, is also an important step in dealing with difficult scenarios.

When someone suggests dinner or a fishing trip, you need to ask of yourself, "Is this medicine?" When someone requests alternative therapy or something that's not familiar, you need to ask, "What's good medicine here?" When Gordon considered the requests of difficult patients—the bulk of his former referral practice—he had two primary guidelines: Never compromise care. Never speak of things he doesn't know about. No matter how reasonable the request, Gordon's response went something like this:

"Mr Jones, I am trained to look for diseases and treat them. I don't really know anything about chelation. What I know comes from the medical literature. I don't claim that it explains everything but what I know about chelation indicates that it isn't helpful and I'm not comfortable recommending it in your particular case. If that is something that you are hoping that I would do, I think we need to talk about it more."

Exit Stage Right

As in any drama, you may be playing a final scene with your difficult patient that has one of you exiting the encounter, perhaps prematurely from your point of view. For no matter how much you try to communicate with this person, impediments to your conversations always seem to bring you back to the same impasse: "I don't want to have that test." "I don't want to take that medicine." "I don't want to see that specialist." Granted, you want to give it your best effort, maybe even suggesting to this person that the scenes between the two of you have become too rough to play:

"This isn't going the way I thought it should go. I wonder how you feel about it." or

"I can see, Mr Jones, that this isn't going the way you had expected. How can I help; what can we do differently together?"

But the reality is that even when you're a great physician, capable of Tony Award performances, you can't please all of the critics all of the time. In fact, sometimes physicians erroneously believe that there are no resistant patients, when, in fact, some are just impossible to direct and simply want to take their cues from someone else.

Who won't relate to the Milwaukee internist whose patient found a Mayo Clinic specialist more to his liking even after awarding her a plaque for her considerable skills. She had kept his high blood pressure under control for a year after others seemingly failed in their attempts. But when the medication was no longer effective, he disappeared. The next she heard was a phone call announcing that his new physician had prescribed a drug that *really* worked. Why hadn't other physicians done the same?

Today the plaque sits in the physician's car trunk. Yet it's still an apt reminder that not every difficult situation is a product of ineffective communication. Sometimes, no matter how devoted or good you are, you become the villain. And sometimes, if the patient doesn't exit first, you simply must relinquish your role. Of course, before you jettison someone from your rolls, you need to make sure you're in compliance with the Americans with Disabilities Act since the very patient who's causing you problems may be covered by this law. Once you know your standing, you can deliver the message:

"I don't think I can work with you any further. We need to talk about how to transfer your care to another provider."

Even when you decide a referral is best for you both, this person may not be out of your life, especially if the new physician is in your practice. Better to be like the

Georgia family physician who made arrangements with the internist across the street to take his patients when he reached an impasse. It worked because both he and his colleague, for whom he returned the favor, knew that quality care was provided in each office.

You may be able to find such an understudy. But your first choice should be a long run for both you and your patient. Granted, you may have little control over the performance of this individual. But you do have control over your own. Recognize that the greatest communication task you face in any medical drama is not simply asking questions or exchanging dialogue. It's understanding the motivations—feelings and behaviors—that drive every human interaction and, in this case, every encounter or scene.

Once you've learned how to harness your thoughts and actions, you'll have new energy to give to your roles as both actor and director. You may not be aiming for bows and a curtain call in difficult situations, but your patients may surprise you. You just may just get a round of applause.

Bibliography

Anstett R. The difficult patient and the physician-patient relationship. *J Fam Pract*. 1980;11:281-286.

Beckman H. Difficult patients. In: Feldman MD, Christensen, JF, eds. *Behavioral Medicine in Primary Care: A Practical Guide*. Stamford, Conn: Appleton & Lange, 1997:20-29.

Crutcher J, Bass M. The difficult patient and the troubled physician. *J Fam Pract*. 1980;11:933-938.

Epstein R, Campbell T, Cohen-Cole S, McWhinney I, Smilkstein G. Perspectives on patient-doctor communication. *J Fam Pract*. 1993;37:377-388.

Freiden R, Lazerson A. Terminating the physician-patient relationship in primary care. *JAMA*. 1979;241:819-822.

Gerard TJ, Riddell JD. Difficult patients: black holes and secrets. *BMJ*. 1988;297:530-532.

Gorlin R, Zucker H. Physicians' reactions to patients: a key to teaching humanistic medicine. *N Engl J Med*. 1983;308:1059-1063.

Groves J. Taking care of the hateful patient. *N Engl J Med*. 1978;298:883-887.

Hahn S, Kroenke K, Spitzger R, et al. The difficult patient: prevalence, psychopathology and functional impairment. *J Gen Intern Med*. 1996;11:1-7.

Irons R. The seductive patient. *Ala Med, J Med Assoc State Ala 64*. 1994;No. 6:13-17.

Kuch J, Schuman S, Curry H. The problem patient and the problem doctor or do quacks make crocks? *J Fam Pract*. 1977;5:647-653.

Lechky O. There are easy ways to deal with difficult patients. *Can Med Assoc J*. 1992;146:1793-1795.

Lin E, Katon W, Von Korff M, et al. Frustrating patients: physician and patient perspectives among distressed high users of medical services. *J Gen Intern Med*. 1991;6:241-246.

McDaniel S, Campbell TL, Seaburn DB. *Family-Oriented Primary Care*. New York, NY: Springer-Verlag New York; 1990.

Mengel M. Physician ineffectiveness due to family-of-origin issues. *Fam Syst Med*. 1987;5:176-190.

Novack D, Suchman A, Clark W, Epstein R, Najberg E, Kaplan C, for the Working Group on Promoting Physician Personal Awareness, American Academy on Physician and Patient. Calibrating the physician: personal awareness and effective patient care. *JAMA*. 1997;278:502-509.

O'Dowd TC. Five years of heartsink patients in general practice. *BMJ*. 1988;297:528-530.

Sharpe M, Mayou R, Seagroatt V, et al. Why do doctors find some patients difficult to help? *Q J Med*. 1994;87:187-193.

Slocum H. Not him again! Thoughts on coping with irritating elderly patients. *Geriatrics 44*. 1989;No. 10:75-84.

Smith S. Dealing with the difficult patient. *Postgrad Med J*. 1995;71:653-657.

Suchman A, Markakis K, Beckman H, Frankel R. A model of empathic communication in the medical interview. *JAMA*. 1997;277:678-682.

Zinn W. Doctors have feelings too. *JAMA*. 1988;259:3296-3298.

Chapter 7

The Substance-abusing Patient: Recognize the Signals

"I accidentally flushed my pills down the toilet."

"Someone stole my purse, which contained my prescription."

"I'm in town overnight on business but my luggage got lost and I don't have my medication."

Do these "excuses" sound eerily familiar? It's likely you've encountered such patients in your practice—those who spell relief with scheduled or controlled substances. Such "drug-seeking" patients are less interested in the therapeutic potential of their prescription and more interested in its other effects. And, say many experts, they'll often stop at nothing to get their drug of choice. In fact, their modus operandi is what makes these particular patients a challenge for physicians. Yes, they'll tell stories about flushed pills, stolen purses, or lost luggage. But they also frequently show up at walk-in clinics on weekends, where no one knows them. Or they may schedule their visit on the day you're covering your colleague's practice.

Whether they're from the community or just passing through town, these individuals show a remarkable ability to spin tales about health problems—often involving pain so acute that only a scheduled drug will give them immediate relief, or so they insist. They may be so skilled at faking an illness—putting blood in their urine to suggest, for example, a recurrence of kidney stones—that you treat the symptoms rather than scheduling a diagnostic procedure. No matter what the ailment, they often even go so far as to tell you which medication works for them.

"There was a drug I got last time that seemed to help. It was called 'Perco'-something," they may innocently suggest. Whether the drug is percocet or morphine, these substance-abusing patients get what they crave by exploiting physicians who are unaware of their intent. No matter how skilled you are as an interviewer, if this person is unknown to you, it's that much harder to evaluate the situation.

Reverting to stereotypes won't help either because there's no single profile that fits. You may think that when it comes to drugs, the only people you have to look out for are those with track marks on their bodies. Yet experts point out that hard core users of heroin or cocaine comprise a relatively small segment of the substance-abusing population that physicians typically see.

The more problematic group physicians face is those who solicit narcotic medication or tranquilizers, often under the guise of medical problems. These people aren't suffering from a disease; or, if they are, they hustle one physician after another (sometimes as many as 20 a day) to obtain drugs for their euphoric effects or even resale.

Some experts also identify drug-seeking patients as those seeking genuine relief from chronic pain or emotional distress. These people, they suggest, are undertreated in the first place, largely because of prevalent fears physicians have about how to best prescribe controlled substances. These fears are tied to unfamiliarity with such drugs.

In any case, you can't spot substance abusers by their profession, race and ethnicity, or even age. They may be businessmen in designer suits or soccer moms in jogging togs. They may wear canvas knapsacks or carry leather briefcases. Whether they're professional or blue-collar, wealthy, poor, or middle class, they're a problem in the making unless you pick up on the signals that they need this drug for more than its therapeutic benefits.

"These patients are smart enough to know how to maximize their chances and thereby put together some medically plausible story," says Edward Senay, MD, retired University of Chicago Pritzker School of Medicine professor and expert in the field. "It's kind of a dance on both sides."

A Bag of Tricks

There is ample evidence that over time most physicians will be confronted by some patients with this problem. Yet not every clinician in every community will encounter drug-seeking individuals. It's possible you could go through your entire career and never come across a single patient who's inappropriate in his or her drug requests. However, it's also possible that you'll face a constant barrage, particularly if you practice in a big city where people don't have far to roam between physicians.

In any case, your ability to deal with these individuals depends largely on your own cunning in spotting them. You'll be less of a target if you're alert to clues and use proper prescribing habits to thwart their efforts. Drug-seeking patients are more likely to manipulate physicians who prescribe without taking an adequate history and doing both physical and laboratory examinations.

While "drug shoppers" use many ploys, they generally fall into four categories, according to Senay, writing in *Psychoactive Drugs: Improving Prescribing Practices*:

- *Transient patients* are frequently out-of-towners whose description of their pain usually differs vastly from its reality. If you suspect such a disparity, a further clue is their demand that you respond with an immediate prescription.

- *Manipulative patients* frequently study the physician as intently as the physician studies them. They draw suspicion because they aren't behaving like typical patients in an ordinary interaction; they're far more intense.

- *Spellbinding patients* or "con" men and women possess powers of persuasion that go beyond what is seen in normal clinical encounters. Often suffering from syndromes such as Munchhausen's or feigning illness, they raise skepticism with their high drama.

- *Coercive patients* use a variety of psychological techniques, from subtle guilt trips to blatant threats of violence, to reach their ends. Physicians who succumb to these tactics usually report that they were aware of the patient's ploys but wanted to "avoid trouble."

In any case, when it comes to drugs, the best way to respond to the ambiguity of any clinical situation is to be knowledgeable about the substances you're prescribing. You'll be inundated with new medication choices every day, and you'll certainly want to try many of them—especially if the pharmaceutical reps have their way. But good prescribing practices are based on predictable drug performances, which you'll only learn through experience.

In other words, you can't possibly know all of the barbiturates, antidepressants, or benzodiazepines out there. But by developing some familiarity with how certain drugs from any one class affect various patients in your practice, you will acquire a solid base from which to critically evaluate any new drugs that come along.

Unfortunately, suggests Senay, many physicians are like compulsive shoppers in that they try to stay current with the latest "styles" in drugs. Instead, they should amass a store of experience with certain medications. That way they'll have a better grasp of the drugs' clinical applications and won't inadvertently contribute to a patient's drug misuse.

Senay recalls, for example, consulting with a prominent psychopharmacologist who was concerned that his elderly father was "drunk" on Valium when it was introduced as a wonder drug in the 1960s. It was only after Senay suggested reducing the dosage by half that his patient was able to experience its therapeutic benefits without any goofy behavior. Not only was Senay's directive right on the mark, it also anticipated the subsequent medical confirmation that Valium's biotransformation is slower in older patients. "Drugs are tricky," says Senay. "If you can use ones that you know and are pretty confident of, then you'll be more efficient and effective."

The Best Defense

Being comfortable with your own prescribing habits is only part of the challenge. A good way to respond when you're not familiar with a patient —or aren't sure of his or her motives—is to offer enough medication for 24 hours, but then insist on a follow-up. Simply explain that you need time to request their medical records and to do additional physical, or even psychiatric, examinations to ensure there's real urgency. If this person is in genuine need, you'll rarely hear an objection. But if he or she is a true manipulator, you'll see real resistance to getting only a day's dosage until further assessment. This patient might very well take flight once he or she senses that their hidden agenda won't be met.

Yet it might not be enough to merely break up the game. Some experts suggest you should be prepared to conduct a substance-abuse history, especially with patients you don't know but suspect as either at-risk or already using drugs inappropriately.

Writing in *Behavioral Medicine in Primary Care*, author Michael Fleming, MD, suggests a general screening framework for all major mood-altering drugs (nicotine, alcohol, prescriptive medications, and illicit drugs) based on a treatment protocol developed for the *National Cancer Institute's Physician Guide*. It reminds physicians to:

- **Ask:** Employ questions that focus on consumption or use self-administered tests to screen for substance use.

- **Assess:** Determine evidence of both physical dependence and other substance-related problems, such as mood-altering drugs or medical and psychiatric disorders.

- **Advise:** Remind this patient of the consequences of continued use and assess his or her readiness to change.

- **Assist:** Help the patient make these changes through written agreements to correct the problem or through referral to a treatment program.

The goal is to identify and deal with the patient's problem, no matter what your approach. Senay would have physicians incorporate a mental status examination along with the diagnostic interview because the two areas are often so inextricably bound. Substance-abuse patterns suggest that people often are not only dependent on multiple drugs but have mental conditions as well. Seeking specific information about the person's personal and family history, along with current behavior and cognitive ability, can help pinpoint additional mood, anxiety, or antisocial personality disorders that may complicate the issue.

Even a basic substance-abuse history helps evaluate the extent of the problem by focusing on particulars, such as the age when the person first used drugs and the point at which his or her usage was the heaviest. This information, as well as relevant data on dosage increases, provides a prognostic framework.

A wide variety of standardized instruments—such as the Michigan Alcoholism Screening Test (MAST) and its spin-off, the Drug Abuse Substance Test (DAST)—produce reliable results based on quantitative measures from a restricted set of questions.

But these tests have their limitations, say some experts. They don't necessarily cover all substances. They may be too long and complex for an initial screening. And they may interfere with the patient-physician interaction because the physician may be more focused on the instrument than on the patient.

The CAGE questionnaire, for instance, is a widely accepted screening tool that relies on four basic questions to explore a patient's use of alcohol:

"Have you ever felt the need to Cut *down on your drinking?"*

"Have you ever felt Annoyed *by criticism of your drinking?"*

"Have you had Guilty *feelings about your drinking?"*

"Have you ever taken a morning Eye *opener?"*

The CAGE has the benefits of being brief and relatively nonconfrontational, yet its drawback is that it is limited to alcohol use. Another test, the Addiction Severity Index (ASI), focuses on both alcohol and drugs. But it's a somewhat structured interview designed to address the severity of problems in areas affected by the patient's abuse, such as marriage and employment.

Physicians will get better responses, Senay believes, if they focus their questions on a core set of 11 substances rather than limiting their inquiry to the standard query, "Do you use drugs or alcohol?" In other words, histories are more accurate when clinicians target questions specifically on central nervous system depressants (barbiturates and benzodiazepines); stimulants (amphetamines, cocaine, cocaine "base" crack); opioids (heroin, codeine, methadone); hallucinogens (lysergic acid diethylamide, methylenodioxyam-hetamine, mescaline); PCP (arylcyclohexylamines); cannabis (pot or hashish); inhalants (paint and glue); nicotine; alcohol; caffeine; and over-the-counter sedatives.

Substance-abuse screening will net more accurate results if you formulate the preliminaries within the context of general health questions and ask them in a manner that's nonjudgmental, empathic, and respectful. It is important to impress on your patient that you want this information because it's integral to assessment of his or her overall well-being. You can introduce the premise by saying:

> *"I'm going to ask some questions now that are rather personal, but for a thorough medical history I have to know certain information."* or
>
> *"I have no reason to suspect any abuse of drugs or alcohol. I'm just trying to know more about your lifestyle so I can take good care of you."*

Reassurance reduces wariness and reinforces that your job is to care for your patient's whole health. Yes, delving into the prospect of substance abuse may seem a daunting task. But it's a necessary one if you're to discover who needs further assessment, advice, and assistance. As Senay observes:

> These days I would say it would border on criminal negligence not to be detecting people who are using substances, especially younger people who may be rescued from "careers" with drugs. And if you explain what you're doing, it doesn't bother the doctor-patient relationship.

Bibliography

Clark W. Effective interviewing and intervention for alcohol problems. In: Lipkin M Jr, Putnam SM, Lazare A, eds. *The Medical Interview: Clinical Care, Education, and Research.* New York, NY: Springer-Verlag New York; 1995:284-293.

Cleary P, Miller M, Bush B, Warburg M, Delbanco, Aronson M. Prevalence and recognition of alcohol abuse in a primary care population. *Am J Med.* 1988;85:466-470.

Collier M. The art of communicating with patients who use alcohol or other drugs. *Md Med J.* 1994;43: 18-21.

Coulehan J, Zettler-Segal M, Block M, McClelland M, Schulberg H. Recognition of alcoholism and substance abuse in primary care patients. *Arch Intern Med.* 1987;147:349-352.

Fleming M, Lawton B, Baier Manwell L, Johnson K, London R. Brief physician advice for problem alcohol drinkers: a randomized controlled trial in community-based primary care practices. *JAMA.* 1997;277:1039-1045.

Kamerow D, Pincus H, MacDonald D. Alcohol abuse, other drug abuse and mental disorders in medical practices: prevalence, costs, recognition and treatment. *JAMA.* 1986;255:2054-2057.

Levinson W, Roter D, Mulloooly J, Dull V, Frankel R. Physician-patient communication: the relationship with malpractice claims among primary care physicians, surgeons. *JAMA.* 1997;277:553-559.

Senay E. Diagnostic interview and mental status examination. In: Lowinson JH, Ruiz P, Millman RB, Langrod JG, eds. *Substance Abuse: A Comprehensive Textbook.* 3rd ed. Baltimore, Md: Williams & Wilkins; 1997:364-369.

Senay E, Schuster C. Principles of rational prescribing. In: Ghodse H, Khan I, eds. *Psychoactive Drugs: Improving Prescribing Practices.* New York NY: World Health Organization; 1988:36-41.

Wallace P. Coping with patients' problems drinking. *Pract.* 1989;233:475-480.

Chapter 8

Common Mental Illnesses: Connect Mind and Body

A medical interview is the best road map clinicians have in determining if patients are suffering from mental illness or other emotional distress. Depression. Panic disorders. The signs are frequently etched on the faces, emitting from the voices, and ingrained in the demeanor of individuals who walk into your office,

Throughout your medical career—especially if you're in primary care—you'll see any number of anxiety, mood, substance abuse, and eating, as well as personality disorders. These conditions can be as crippling to patients—and as perplexing to physicians—as other physical ailments.

Unfortunately, clinicians don't always pick up on the verbal and nonverbal cues— the tearful eyes, laden speech, or sad disposition—indicating a myriad of problems. Some statistics suggest that physicians fail to identify 50% to 75% of patients suffering from common mental disorders.

Clinicians, suggests Robert L. Spitzer, MD, in a December 14, 1994, *Journal of the American Medical Association*, are hampered by a lack of sufficient knowledge of diagnostic criteria and an uncertainty about which questions to ask in evaluating those standards. In addition, many of them are so driven by the hurried pace of today's office practice that they forget to do a proper interview.

"Too many physicians don't even look at the patient while they're getting a history," says Alan Enelow, MD, coauthor of the book *Interviewing and Patient Care*. "They don't make eye contact. Managed care has forced many physicians to dispose of patients rapidly so they can get on to the next one. There isn't a chance to really look at this person."

Despite those drawbacks, interviews remain the focal point in assessing anyone's mental status. By building rapport—even in a managed care environment—you can facilitate conversation so patients feel free to talk about what's troubling them.

But good interviewing, particularly to detect mental illness, is more than just figuring out the right question to ask or the best time to ask it. It's more than having your queries so well crafted and well paced that you could complete the process with a computer.

Instead, it's returning to the "art of medicine"—getting to know the person behind the patient. In fact, paying attention to each individual—using your own powers of observation along with a few well-placed open-ended statements—can take you down new roads that need exploring:

"What brings you here today?" or

"What troubles are you having?"

Your query may not yield an immediate admission. But that doesn't mean your observations are incorrect. Rather, it's just a sign along the roadside that this patient isn't ready to make the connection and you need to continue the journey by encouraging him or her to tell more of his or her story.

At the same time, you're poised to observe landmarks—signs and symptoms—along the way: weight loss, low energy, an emptiness in the eyes. You might just see something in a face or manner that suggests deeper troubles. In any case, once you identify the source, it's a natural next step to say:

"Now you've told me this, this, and this. You look depressed to me. Tell me what you think."

If you've built sufficient trust, that should be enough to break down any inhibitions or denials by this person. Patients won't hide their angst, suggest some experts, if they've seen that their physician makes eye contact, pays attention, and looks empathetic.

Even when the patient begins to cry during the interview, you don't have to shy away from the situation, writes Enelow. Instead, such a release can be helpful. A person who is fighting tears may not be able to speak. But an individual who weeps openly may find enough relief to resume talking.

Yet clinicians often make the error, in their discomfort, of interrupting patients with supportive remarks before these individuals have a chance to "cry out" their pain. Instead, physicians should maintain a "sympathetic silence" until the tears have stopped and they can resume the interview. In the meantime, the important move is to be supportive with:

"You must be feeling very bad."

If this same patient is on the verge of tears, as Enelow suggests, which is making it difficult for him or her to speak, you might want to create the opportunity to cry by confronting the issue:

"You look like you are about to cry."

Picking Up on Panic Disorder

Most of us will experience the abrupt and intense symptoms of a panic attack at some time in our lives. As distressing as these episodes may be, they're usually brief and aren't life-threatening. But at least 3 million Americans have panic disorder, a major anxiety condition dominated by a series of attacks that recur with such frequency that one avoids activities. Panic disorder has a variety of complex causes, including genetics or developmental or life experiences.

If patients are diagnosed correctly and treated or referred appropriately, the medications—benzodiazepines—can make dramatic improvements. Panic disorder is often symptomatic of other debilitating psychiatric conditions (among them agoraphobia, the fear of open and crowded places).

Whatever the root, the symptoms—from flushes and chills to fear of dying—are so sudden and severe that they often scare patients into seeing their physicians. Perhaps you've treated someone like the young woman who came in after a powerful episode in the supermarket. Overwhelmed by the fear that the end was near, she ran from the checkout line to her car and sped home.

Or maybe your colleague surprises you with the same sense of impending doom. Lanny Copeland, MD, president of the American Academy of Family Physicians and vice president of primary care development for Phoebe Putney Health Systems in Albany, Georgia, remembers his surprise at finding a friend in the emergency room suffering from symptoms that the surgeon could only explain with, "I thought I was going to die."

Feelings of doom are a frequent marker for a disorder that can cause physical or somatic symptoms and other behaviors. Patients report racing hearts and an inability to get their breath. They complain of nausea, faintness, or even chest pain. They hyperventilate. They tremble, tingle, or say they feel numb. They even experience preoccupation and fright along with a sense of detachment and fog.

Whatever their complaints, these individuals provide readily observable clues. You'll see the foot that swings and fingers that tap incessantly, or you'll hear about the symptoms that could add up to an anxiety disorder or other condition. In fact, to pick up on the cues of any emotional or mental disorder, you should pay close attention to this person's habitus, noting his or her facial expressions and demeanor and watching how he or she sits and moves.

Unfortunately, says Enelow, too often physicians focus on the chart in taking a history, when they should look at the individual. They pay more attention to words on a page and less to the psycho-physiological symptoms in front of them. They may not see the demeanor—droop of the shoulders or low level of energy—that could indicate depression. They may not catch the significance when this person suggests, "Gee, I feel funny being here this morning talking to you about the symptoms I've been having."

In fact, as this patient reels off a description of what's bothering him or her, a story might emerge with enough information to make a diagnosis without taking extra time or scheduling unnecessary testing. Or there's enough evidence in the person's habitus to change the direction of your questioning. For example, behavioral signs may suggest an opening:

"You look very tense to me."

Whatever wording you choose, the idea is to describe to this person something that you find striking about his or her behavior. Called confrontation, the ploy, which Enelow describes, spotlights demeanors that this individual may be dimly aware of—or not aware of at all. It has use in many situations, particularly when you're trying to find the root of an emotion:

"You seem frightened." or

"You sound angry."

In any case, such a statement is likely to change the direction of the conversation, bringing into focus topics that your patient may not think of or be inclined to address. By confronting this person, you're giving him or her an opportunity to move beyond the discomfort of the situation, at least enough to talk about how he or she feels.

Incidentally, confrontation in a medical interview shouldn't have the same emotional or hostile overtones of confrontation in everyday conversation. Instead, your own demeanor should reflect what Enelow calls a "sympathetic interest." Granted, your irritation may call attention to this person's behavior. But it's your concern in finding what's behind the tension or tears that should be expressed here.

Detecting Depression

When Copeland practiced family medicine in a small, rural community 40 miles away from the nearest psychiatrist, he was definitely the gatekeeper in flagging patients with depression. Over time, he became adept in identifying the illness, hearing again and again about blue spells, sleeping difficulties, and general lack of interest. Or he heard it in the comments:

"You know I just don't feel right. I just really feel down."

Nevertheless, at even a hint of suspicion, the family physician would question how his patient was feeling or how long he or she had suffered the symptoms of a condition suffered by 18 million Americans.

Epidemiological studies suggest a lifetime prevalence of the most severe form, major depression, in 7% to 12% of men and 20% to 25% of women, making it an important issue in both public health and office-based medicine. Further, in primary care settings there's a 5% to10% prevalence, with a higher rate in people who have other medical problems, such as Parkinson's disease and stroke.

Depression is triggered by complex genetic, biochemical, behavioral, social, cultural, and developmental causes. While such drugs as antibiotics and antihypertensives can also stimulate episodes, so can life's stressors—loss of a parent, spouse, relationship, job, or self-esteem. No matter what the source, however, the proof of the problem, as with panic disorder, is often in the patient's presentation.

"The absolute point is that physicians have to show empathy," says Copeland. "If we aren't going to listen, we've really done the patient a disservice. There's a sense of accomplishment when you can reassure someone that you are there to help and there is medication and treatment that will help them."

Nonetheless, you may get your first clue in a visceral reaction to this person and his or her behavior. Perhaps you'll feel sympathy at your patient's suffering or you'll become anxious because he or she seems jumpy. Maybe you'll even share this individual's sadness.

He or she may complain of insomnia or other sleep disorders, as well as either weight or appetite gains and losses. You may see the hopelessness in his or her lackluster eyes. Or you'll hear it in a low tone of voice or in a speech pattern that has slowed precipitously to include only a few words.

Fatigue and loss of energy may be apparent in his or her manner, posture, and thinking. He or she may have trouble concentrating, making decisions, or volunteering information, which can make your task in collecting information even more challenging.

Further, depression begets a general lack of interest or pleasure in activities and an overall sense of feeling worthless. Apathy. Guilt. They're part of a syndrome that can have as its center low self-esteem and profound feelings of emptiness or loneliness, which may even lead to recurrent thoughts of suicide.

In any case, the number and intensity of symptoms vary with the severity of the condition. On one end of the spectrum are simple anxiety and mood swings signifying mild depression. On the other end are a multitude of indicators of major or more severe depressive illness. The signs for the latter can become so pronounced as the disease progresses that a patient might be totally withdrawn, even spending his or her day huddled in bed.

Depression is considered major if an individual exhibits a variety of symptoms, including persistent depressed mood or pervasive loss of interest in living. It's minor when the condition is prompted by an event, such as divorce or job loss, which causes functional impairment exceeding normal expectations.

Any level of depression will be missed if a physician doesn't practice routine screening. In fact, the interview itself might bring some relief for symptoms of mild to moderate depression, which is easily treated. Because the hallmark of major depression is a lack of capacity for pleasure, physicians would do well, write Steven A. Cole, MD, and his colleagues in *Behavioral Medicine in Primary Care*, to focus their initial questions on:

"What do you do for a good time?" and

"How is your sleep?"

Despite the patient's focus on other physical complaints or even denial that a problem exists, these queries often yield the kind of information necessary to diagnose depression. Today's clinicians have a variety of other potentially effective diagnostic tools. Among them is PRIME-MD (Primary Care Evaluation of Mental Disorders), a standardized, brief, and easy assessment procedure that facilitates rapid and accurate diagnoses.

PRIME-MD focuses on five of the most common mental disorders identified by the *Diagnostic and Statistical Manual of Mental Disorders*, 4th ed. (DSM-IV). PRIME-MD highlights mood, anxiety, and somatoform conditions, as well as possible alcohol abuse/dependence and eating problems. While other screening scales suggest the likelihood of a mental disorder, PRIME-MD also confirms it.

Patients fill out a one-page questionnaire highlighting symptoms in five diagnostic areas. "Yes" answers for any of the 26 questions sends physicians into a more detailed interview from specific modules outlined in an accompanying guide. Yielding a variety of information, PRIME-MD has proved a useful tool in office-based settings because of it's reliability, specificity, and efficiency.

In recognizing depression, physicians also should be cognizant of other mental, anxiety, and personality disorders, as well as dementia, substance abuse, and general medical conditions that can be easily confused with it. With symptoms that are often similar, the conditions also may be interrelated.

Similarly, knowing barriers in recognizing depression can help you and your patient overcome them, writes Cole. Specifically, patients may actually present with somatic problems such as pain, fatigue, and insomnia that aren't recognized as depression. Physicians may worry that they're opening up "Pandora's Box" by paying attention to emotional issues, when managing such problems can conserve resources.

Both patients and physicians may also be stymied by the stigma that still exists with an illness that is really no different from other chronic diseases such as hypertension and diabetes. In fact, a communication priority must be to explain to both patients and families that depression is a treatable medical illness.

"You don't put people on antidepressive medication and say see you in two months," says Copeland. "You talk to them about the ongoing visits and how long they'll be taking their medications and the side effects. They're much better educated patients when they know what to expect down the pike."

And the payoffs can be long-lasting for you both. Copeland says some of the most grateful patients have been those whose depression he's recognized, diagnosed, and treated.

He recalls the phone call one Sunday evening from a distraught medical colleague who asked to come to see him. When the internist arrived, he described a pattern Copeland had seen all too frequently in patients: lack of sleep, a sense of worthlessness, feelings of being down.

The visit lasted only an hour, but Copeland saw his colleague in a follow-up office appointment and started him on medication. He immediately felt better. Years later, the man's wife sought out the physician at a function and gave him a comment that still prompts goose bumps.

"She said, 'I want you to thank you for what you did for my husband by recognizing his illness. He still takes his medication. I know this sounds heroic, but you saved his life.'"

Bibliography

Cole S, Christensen J, Raju M, Feldman M. Depression. In: Feldman MD, Christensen JF, eds. *Behavioral Medicine in Primary Care: A Practical Guide*. Stamford, Conn: Appleton & Lange; 1997:177-192.

Enelow A, Forde D, Brummel-Smith K. *Interviewing and Patient Care*. 9th ed. New York, NY: Oxford University Press; 1996.

Feder A, Robbin S. Personality disorders. In: Feldman MD, Christensen JF, eds. *Behavioral Medicine in Primary Care: A Practical Guide*. Stamford, Conn: Appleton & Lange; 1997:20-29.

Levinson W, Engel C. Anxiety. In: Feldman MD, Christensen JF, eds. *Behavioral Medicine in Primary Care: A Practical Guide*. Stamford, Conn: Appleton & Lange; 1997:20-29.

Mance R, Cohen-Cole S. Interviewing the psychotic patient. In: Lipkin M Jr, Putnam SM, Lazare A, eds. *The Medical Interview: Clinical Care, Education, and Research*. New York, NY: Springer-Verlag New York; 1995:275-283.

Spitzer R, Williams J, Kroenke K, et al. Utility of a new procedure for diagnosing mental disorders in primary care: the PRIME-MD 1000 study. *JAMA*. 1992;272:1749-1756.

Strain J, Putman S, Goldberg R. The mental status examination. In: Lipkin M Jr, Putnam SM, Lazare A, eds. *The Medical Interview: Clinical Care, Education, and Research*. New York, NY: Springer-Verlag New York; 1995:83-103.

Index

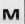
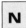

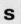